Slender Threads

a young person's guide to Parkinson's Disease

Pete Langman

Published by Pete Langman, 2013.

www.petelangman.com

ISBN-13: 978-0-957-5662-0-0

To my basal ganglia.
R.I.P.

CONTENTS

Acknowledgements

This book has been a trial to write, and at times has felt nigh-on impossible. I owe a debt of gratitude to several people, without whom I would never have begun, let alone finished.

Colleen Henderson-Heywood stands apart in many ways, not least through her having been a constant source of encouragement and a valuable touchstone for my thoughts throughout the writing and editing process. It is also fair to point out that this book was pretty much her idea.

Others have read, commented, corrected and cajoled me when I needed it most. Sometimes they've shouted at me, too. Uppermost amongst these, and in alphabetical order, are Angela Brand, Kay Diggens, Harvey Guest, Rachel Junior, Karen Johnson, Jacqueline Johnson, Rebekah Kortokraks, Randell McLeod, and Jon Stamford.

Dr. Jon Stamford is also due thanks for his fine work in correcting my medical faux pas.

The good people at Parkinson's UK and the Cure Parkinson's Trust.

My deepest thanks are reserved for Cathy Relf, whose editorial skills and unique take on the subject matter improved this book beyond measure.

Prologue

OK. Where to start?

It seems the height of arrogance to say 'I'm writing a book on Parkinson's Disease', but I am. This is it. I have begun. What happens next is, at this moment in time, something of a mystery. It's December 13th 2011, 6.09am, and I've been awake since about ten past four. I don't sleep much any more. I'm propped up in bed nursing an injured shoulder that was operated on two days ago, so I ought to be focused on that. But, since January 2008, my focus has been on my PD, and how it has progressively changed me. It's a progressive condition, so it's only right that it should.

On the day I was diagnosed, I failed to take in exactly what it meant, and I still have. That's because it means something different every day. Every day it affects me in a different way, a new way, a worse way, a better way. My relationship with PD started before my diagnosis: diagnosis just gave me an idea of the destination. I already had an inkling of the means of transport. And that's exactly where I am now with this book. I know what it will say, but I don't know how it will say it, or in what order. This book will be as much a new experience for me as it will be for you, the reader. I suspect that keeping that in mind will help when it fails to make sense. That's what I do. Sometimes the PD does stuff I don't expect and, well, there's only one thing to do: put your hands in the air, intone 'whatever', and roll with it.

I don't expect you to enjoy this, but I think you might just appreciate it. If you're reading because you have just been diagnosed, well, good luck; if it's because someone you know and love has been diagnosed, well, good luck.

This book is designed for a number of different audiences. Its primary aim is to give you, the newly diagnosed, and you, the friends and family of the newly diagnosed some idea of what it might be like to live with this irritating disease. Hopefully, it will help. It is not intended to answer technical questions, medical questions, or anything of that ilk, though it will necessarily consider such things as it trundles past them.

I'm primarily interested in how this disease makes us feel, how it affects us psychologically. In order to achieve this I often stray into what feels like memoir territory. It may seem at points as if I am writing simply for myself, my family and friends, my lovers. Well, I am. But to me the only way of communicating something useful is to talk about how it made me feel. I only hope that by writing honestly and openly (or, at least, trying to), I can help others to find their own way of dealing with this disease. If I drift off into some reverie or other (and I will), bear with me – it may seem unconnected but there is a point to it all. To know how we are affected, we need to know who we are. Parkinson's has taught me a lot about who I am; some of it's been good, some of it not so good.

I have chosen the hook on which to hang this work somewhat arbitrarily … after all, it appears that I was chosen arbitrarily by the thing I mean to hang. People are, as the Renaissance philosopher Francis Bacon noted, temperamentally predisposed to seeing order where there is none – this is why we have religion, science, superstition, conspiracy theories (as he was the subject of my PhD, I spent rather a lot of time with this particular gentleman). The very idea that something as complex and beautiful as, say, the eye, or as daftly exotic as a bird of paradise, has come about through a series of random mutations in which the most fit (as in fitting, rather than physically well-conditioned, or even good-looking) animal gets to reproduce and convey its peculiar advantage down its family line is challenging for us. It's much more comforting to think teleologically, that is, to assume that each thing has a purpose, that each thing was designed to fulfil a need, designed with an end-point. That this is why the polar bear is so good at being a polar bear. But nothing is finished. Everything is in a state of flux. It's the way of things. So we impose order.

I, too, have imposed an arbitrary order on things. Well, you've got to start somewhere, right? I've chosen to structure the book around Jacques's 'Seven Ages of Man' speech from *As You Like It*, simply because it gives a natty little title to each chapter, and because Shakespeare does seem to have hit on a pretty good formula. It works for me. And that's all this book purports to be – what works for me, what's happened to me, ultimately, I'm trying to write the book I would have liked to have read four and a half years ago.

All the world's a stage,
And all the men and women merely players;
They have their exits and their entrances,
And one man in his time plays many parts,
His acts being seven ages. At first, the infant,
Mewling and puking in the nurse's arms,
Then the whining schoolboy, with his satchel
And shining morning face, creeping like snail
Unwillingly to school. And then the lover,
Sighing like furnace, with a woeful ballad
Made to his mistress' eyebrow. Then a soldier,
Full of strange oaths and bearded like the pard,
Jealous in honour, sudden and quick in quarrel,

Seeking the bubble reputation
Even in the cannon's mouth. And then the justice,
In fair round belly with good capon lined,
With eyes severe and beard of formal cut,
Full of wise saws and modern instances;
And so he plays his part. The sixth age shifts
Into the lean and slippered pantaloon
With spectacles on nose and pouch on side;
His youthful hose, well saved, a world too wide
For his shrunk shank, and his big manly voice,
Turning again toward childish treble, pipes
And whistles in his sound. Last scene of all,
That ends this strange eventful history,
Is second childishness and mere oblivion,
Sans teeth, sans eyes, sans taste, sans everything.
(*As You Like It*, 2.7.139-67)

I hope that this book helps, if only in some small way.

Good luck.

Slender Threads

Slender Threads

This is a blog post I wrote in the middle of writing this book, on February 23, 2012, which, I think, goes some way to explaining what the hell I'm doing here.

> On such slender threads
> as these are we suspended,
> restrained, or mended

Something like that, anyway. Looking backwards is fraught with danger, as the temptation is to remonstrate with oneself at length over a bad choice, over a missed opportunity, over and above any suspicion of self-congratulation for a difficult decision made well. Writing what is essentially a directed autobiography, the work which I am currently avoiding at seemingly all costs, and which has sent me into a frenzy of adverbial apoplexy, is a dangerous thing for someone prone to such analysis. The book, A Young Person's Guide to Parkinson's, is in large part an attempt to create what I would have loved to have been able to read when I was diagnosed. I may very well not have liked it, let alone enjoyed it, but the idea of a work which traces its fingers over the outlines and creases which PD created and continues to create in one life would, I think, have stood me in good stead.

The problem with it is simple: in writing it, I needs must retrace not only the outlines of the disease, but those of the ripples it sent, and continues to send, through my life. Sometimes, I find myself shaking my head at my idiocy, my arrogance, my breathtaking froideur. At other times, I think I am one of the luckiest people around (within certain parameters). Both feelings are dangerous. Recently, I've struggled to achieve a few things, mostly because I'm working in spite of people who have nothing vested in my success, nor any clear understanding of what form it might take. But for all the dangers of looking back, there are clear lessons to be learnt. My current silence in blog terms is largely due to the intense energy being invested in this project, which, like most of my writing, has an emotional and intellectual event horizon far beyond the singularity of its merely being written. That and the fact that I need a cup of tea. I've been tweaking my shoulder changing light bulbs, panicking about the subsequent pain but finally being assured that it's only to be expected. It hurts now. I suspect that this is because it knows I'm writing about it. In similar fashion, writing about PD enhances and magnifies its symptoms and their accompanying issues. I'm already hyper-aware of my body, so writing about its travails just perks it up. As I cast my mind backwards, whether simply to narrate the order of things, or perhaps to dig through the murkier parts of my past in an attempt to locate those vital moments where the whole thing changed (an impossible task, but one rendered all the more attractive as a result), the futility of reverse engineering becomes ever more apparent.

On Tuesday, I was driving to Bromley (yes! I can finally drive again …), and trundling around the M25 when I heard a loud bang behind me. I looked into my rear view mirror only to see a small car cut directly across the carriageway, at 90 degrees to the direction of traffic. Somehow it managed to avoid the two large lorries which were travelling just behind me at a reasonably healthy lick. Actually, avoid is an utterly misleading word. The lorries simply didn't transform the car into a small pile of twisted metal, and the carriageway into a charnal pit. Having missed the lorries, the car drove directly up the bank at the side of the carriageway, crashed through the fence and into the field. The lorries ground to a halt, and the carriageway remained clear and free-running.

There is no clearer indication of the nature of the past. This all happened two or three car lengths behind me. A matter of, well, less than a second. Had I been travelling a little more slowly, just a tiny bit, the car would have clipped my rear. A tiny bit faster, and I would have been oblivious of the closeness of utter disaster. As it was, only the fence was harmed. I hope.

On such slender threads indeed.

Mewling and puking in the nurse's arms –
on becoming aware of change

It's an odd place to start, as it's already behind you. By the time you are reading this, as the movie ransom notes go, you will already have been diagnosed. You're here because you want to know what's going to happen, what it is you should do, how you ought to react, how to cope. You're here because your consultant speaks a funny language, and, let's face it, you were too freaked out to listen that carefully. Once the word is spoken it grows so big so quickly that nothing else can fit in your head. This, however, is the perfect time to pause, reflect, remember, to go through things that you know. It's time to place both feet firmly on the ground and look at how you got here. Not the mechanism; the path. After all, if you don't know where you've come from, how can you know you're not simply retracing steps when you start on going again?

The disease. What it is.

Parkinson's is a disease of the brain. There are various theories regarding how or why it appears, but they rely on weak inference from statistical data. There are direct correlations between PD and potential exposure to pesticides, and inverse correlations between smoking and Parkinson's. That is, you're more likely to develop Parkinson's if you've been exposed to various pesticides, and less likely if you smoke. But, as they say in statistics classes the length and breadth of the land, correlation does not mean causation. Equally, there are several genes associated with Parkinson's, but on the whole there is not enough data for any direct causative role to be assigned.

The fact is that while the mechanisms of Parkinson's are increasingly being unravelled, the reason or reasons that these mechanisms click into gear are simply a mystery. Parkinson's (or PD, as I shall name it hence), lacks a pathogen. There is no virus, bacterium or parasite that causes it.

It's hard to concoct a simple analogy to explain PD to the non-technicallly minded (such as myself). At its simplest, PD is a disease whose symptoms are caused by a lack of dopamine. Dopamine is a neurotransmitter; that is, a chemical involved in the transmission of nerve signals. It's manufactured by cells in the brain, particularly in the basal ganglia. In people with Parkinson's (hereafter PWP), these cells begin to die, leading to a lack of dopamine, leading to problems with the communication between the brain and the bits. It's then that symptoms appear.

It's obviously far more complex than that, and we'll get into the whys and wherefores as and when (or if and when), it becomes appropriate.

Thus far, my favourite analogies to explain this bit of PD are as follows:

1.   The bad Skype connection. When you're on Skype, and the connection is poor, or the bandwidth low, you can hear before you can see ... and the video is often slow, jumpy, tortuous ... *that's* what it feels like sometimes.

2.   The 10 fps movie camera. A movie is filmed at 35 fps. That means every second, 35 pictures are taken. This makes for a smooth playback. The PWP often works at, say, 10 fps. Slow things look fine, but move

to anything more rapid and the image gets juddery and jittery.

Before I started this book, I'd been writing a blog for a year or so, partially as a way of keeping track of myself. In many ways it's a similar process, except that your audience is utterly different. A blog is instant: it allows you to react to things when they're fresh in your mind, when you can see them clearly. They are read, generally, within a few days of publication, while the reader can imagine the feelings presented as fresh and raw. This, for example, is the last blog post I wrote before launching into this opening chapter (and yes, I know it's taken me over six weeks to move from introduction to chapter one), and it's one that received some interesting responses:

Unexpected side-effects may include [first published 3 Feb, 2012]

After my several weeks of beslingification, I had noticed that my left hand seemed considerably worse in the PD department than once it had been. Weaker. Slower. Stiffer. Shakier. Hang on … shakier? Yes. The tremor seems to have begun. It manifests at, well, sometimes rather inconvenient times. Damn inconvenient times. But it certainly manifests.

This afternoon, I delivered one of what I suspect will be many guitar lessons to a fellow twitterer who just happens to live stateside. Ah, the joys of Skype. The usual stuff, but luckily to someone with an ear, a brain, and some serious motivation. So, nothing too onerous. Yes, my left hand is getting worse, it doesn't quite 'get' the strings perfectly any more. It doesn't quite skim over the fingerboard like a swallow. The notes don't really come out right.

Naturally, at one point I tried to play something to my pupil, and tried a Paco Pena piece I used to know, selecting a bit from the middle which is rather cool. I get to the bit where my third and fourth fingers are on the fifth fret and my first on the second, and a wee judder knocks my fingertips off the strings. Hmm. So I pick up my steel-string, retune it and start to play … with only two fingers on the board it'll be fine, surely? The first knuckle on my second finger starts to collapse and straighten at speed.

This operation seems to have triggered an acceleration of symptomatic decline in my fingers.

The fact is, there are now two more tunes that I can't play. Two more boxes unticked. Two jam jars filled, as a friend of mine pointed out today, with bits of dead me, like Seth Brundle in The Fly. Not only am I falling apart, but I am recording its falling.

This blog is effectively a museum. A museum containing the bits of me which don't work. Eventually there will be more in it than in me.

But by then, it will be too late.

I have an idea of what it's like to read another's blog, but revisiting my own is really rather strange. I sound quite sad, and I wonder how I'd read this were it by someone else. Ultimately, it feels like a particular point in time, preserved. Unfortunately not a particularly pleasant point.

But the book, now the book is a different beast entirely. I edited out three errors in that blog post before copying it over. Errors that are due solely to the fact that my typing is ropey, and that I tend to write and post very quickly. Errors that, while irritating, don't worry me overmuch. Mainly because they're easy to edit out (as I did today) on an ad hoc basis. The book, or the essay, or the article ... well, they're printed on bits of paper, and every mistake, every clumsy piece of prose, every factual error remains, unchanged. They are testament to sloppy thinking, sloppy editing, sloppy, well, everything.

It's more than simply unalterable longevity, however. The book needs to appeal to multiple audiences, separated by time rather than distance, and to multiple readings in a way that a blog post, effectively a 'read it and pass it back' piece of work, does not. When you share a book, it's a personal, physical transaction, an emotional transfer in which the sharer gives as a gift their good name and reputation along with the tangible artefact. When one shares a blog post, one hits the 'share' button, or copies the URL and emails it. There's very little emotional investment going on.

You may currently be wondering what on earth I'm doing talking about the socio-cultural differentiation between blogs and books when presented as gifts. When the PWP is just a P (person), or perhaps PWPBTDK (person with Parkinson's but they don't know), all manner of things happen. It's only retrospectively, following diagnosis or on realising that there really is something wrong, that stuff gets ascribed a value. That is, when you look at something and place the PD flag-on-a-pin firmly in it. That's where you are, I suspect. Scrutinising the past and going 'ah ...' as it becomes obvious why certain of these things happened. Once more, we are desperate to attach meaning to everything.

In a similar way we look back at writings which were conceived in the moment, in the heat of passion, and can view them somewhat more coldly, dispassionately. We can take a step outside ourselves and look in. Whether we like what we see is another matter entirely.

It's quite hard to pinpoint the exact moment that a gradual change began. There are several reasons for this, not least that gradual changes are by their very nature small changes, and at first they are wholly imperceptible. It's difficult to think of an analogy that doesn't involve something overwhelmingly negative, but I guess that's the point. When the gall wasp crawls out of the apple, it's the first visible sign that something has happened, barring your witnessing of the laying of the first egg. Likewise, when the first symptom of PD shows its delightful little head, you can be sure your basal ganglia have been dropping like flies for some time. Furthermore, that first symptom isn't going to be some earth-shattering event, upon whose heels follow the three horsemen of PD – tremor, muscle stiffness and slowness of movement – oh no. It'll be something so subtle, such as your fingers not quite closing properly on something fiddly, that you'll be able to list thirty good, solid reasons for it before getting to PD.

It isn't hard to pinpoint the exact moment that a gradual change began; it's impossible. You won't feel it when it starts, and when you feel it, you'll never guess the cause, unless you're a raging hypochondriac who gets very, very lucky (in terms of Milliganesque Cassandrisms). This means that what we're doing now, scouring our memories for the first symptom so that we can rage against it, is one of our more frustrating reactions. And yet, if we are to attach meaning to this, this failure in our brain, then we need to set the parameters. We need to know the beginnings. Furthermore, if we can't find some sense of the beginning, how do we expect to recognise the end?

To accept something, to assimilate something, to beat something, we need to know where it begins and we end. Me? I don't care. I know there's no beating it. I have no choice but to accept it – because it *is*. As for assimilation, well ... we're best off negotiating with it.

On the way of the empty hand

The first thing that I noticed was my left hand. It was subtle, but then I was doing something that required subtlety. I had taken up karate three or four years previously, for social, self-defence and fitness purposes, and was doing reasonably well. I was very physically fit, thanks to my gym regimen, and could easily compete physically with fellow students ten or more years my junior. I worked very hard, not only practising at home, but pushing myself as hard as I could in the dojo. I advanced, though perhaps not as much as I would have liked.

A lot of karate training is taken up with performing kata, set sequences of moves that form an almost balletic impression of a fight with multiple opponents. As the grades advance, the kata not only become more complex, but the standard to which one must perform them increases. The higher the grade, the sharper, more focused and more accurate the kata must be. The position of the fingers, the angle of the arm, the placement of the feet ... all these must be just so. Kata switch between graceful and balletic moves to swift, powerful, brutal attack and defence: the ethos of karate is one technique, one kill. Kinda. Anyway, both types of move require excellent fine motor control, to stop and start the moves with precision. The moves are then repeated and repeated and repeated.

It started, I think, with my left fist. When performing punches during basic training, the fist is to be kept clenched, cocked, and ready on the hip. It must be pulled back as far as possible, and the elbow tucked in rather than sticking out. Every now and then I'd get 'adjusted'. Naturally, the mode of adjustment varies from sensei to sensei. Some are traditional (read: violent), some more progressive (read: conciliatory). Mine were mostly the latter, though they strayed into traditional territory every now and again. This is a martial art after all.

I began to get adjusted more and more, and, my attention drawn to my left hand, I began to notice other things. During warm-ups, we would open and close our fists at speed, and my left hand seemed a little slower. I, not unreasonably, put this down to years of playing the guitar for eight hours a day. Everything we do comes at a price, and the price of whatever guitaristic skills I possessed was the slow disintegration of my left hand now manifest. Or so I assumed.

Now, I know that this was when it started, the slow road to diagnosis, but when? When did it start?

Which year? Which month? This I cannot say, but were I to hazard a guess, I'd say 2005/6, a full two years before my actual diagnosis, maybe even 2004. There was more, however.

In addition to the minor adjustments to my left fist came something a little more serious, in training terms, anyway, as I began to lose the shape of my kata. It turned out that my ability to perform movements accurately and fast was diminishing in the left hand, which meant that my kata began to look unbalanced, as my left-hand movements became progressively weaker and less accurate than my right. This meant, naturally, that I began to slow down in terms of progress. I graded less regularly, was asked to work on higher grade katas more rarely. Which meant, naturally, that my progress slowed. More importantly, in terms of practising martial arts, I started to get hit more often while sparring. Obviously, getting hit is something of an occupational hazard when you're indulging in such a sport, but there's being hit by someone better, or by someone there or thereabouts who made a better job of that particular exchange, and then there's being hit by someone who has very little right to hit you. This is what started happening.

My left-side defences became porous. The problem was exacerbated as the majority of techniques would come from my opponent's right-hand side, as the majority were right-handed – whether by foot or fist, it would land on my left side. This meant two things. First that my feeble left-hand defence made my opponent's right-hand technique more liable to get through, and secondly, once my weakness in the left side had been established, further assaults would naturally be concentrated in this area. It only took a few weeks of being surprised before it stopped being something I could put down to a bad day, or feeling a bit off. Naturally, I compensated, and generally speaking the trick to not losing a fight is to avoid getting hit. But as my right hand assumed more defensive duties, so it became more difficult to comprehensively win a fight. This, along with the problem of my kata becoming worse rather than better, meant that I fell further behind.

One of the secondary results of this kind of decline is that you begin to feel rather pissed off with it all. You're failing, or regressing, for no apparent reason and it really pisses you off. Well, it pissed me off no end. The gradual deterioration is especially strange when you feel you ought to be improving. You work hard, you practise and train hard, and yet you seem to be on a different timeline to everyone else. They are accelerating in their development while you are slowing down, grinding to a halt, even going backwards.

This regression gradually sapped me of self-confidence, and I started to lose my way, becoming disillusioned with a sport I had enjoyed immensely. I continued to train, but out of bloody-mindedness rather than delight, and I started to search for excuses for my poor performance. Of course, I was entering vicious circle country. But this wasn't the only thing that was misfiring.

On the guitar

Back when I was a young thing, I was a professional guitarist, playing gigs, doing the odd session and managing to gain the accolade of being made Head of Rock Guitar at the Musician's Institute in London. This was not nearly as impressive as it sounds, but wasn't bad at all. In 1995 I nailed myself a monthly tuition column in Guitar and Bass magazine. My thoughts and notes were disseminated from Croydon to China. People were actually reading my words, playing my exercises, gazing admiringly at my byline and doing what I used to do when I was a young guitar player – quietly going 'wow' to themselves, and turning the page. I was on my way to ... well, to a bingo hall in Doncaster, to seventies revival weekends in Pontins ... to the graveyard of ambition. I still remember standing in the dressing room, or security control room as it was, and looking at the stage replete with Christmas tree and Santa in his sled backdrop, then peering at the bolted-down tables our audience were going to sit at during the show, and thinking to myself ... is this it? When I was in my early twenties I'd had my chance to jump on board the bandwagon but been too dumb to notice.

Over the final five years of the 20th century I got so disillusioned with music, the industry and my place in it that I could barely play in front of people. My bloody-mindedness, the quality that had served me so well in my pursuit for guitaristic perfection, simply abandoned me, and I made a quite momentous decision. I retired.

For me, someone who between the ages of fifteen and thirty had practised between four and eight hours a day, every day, it was almost a bereavement. I didn't just get a job to go alongside the guitar playing, or stop being a 'pro'. No, not I. Never one to do things by halves, I simply went cold turkey. I stopped completely. For the first two or three years, I simply didn't touch the instrument. Instead, I poured myself into my new passion, English literature. In 1999 I went to Queen Mary, University of London, to study English. The idea was twofold. Firstly, I was unsure what to do next, so I thought getting a degree would give me three years of legitimately sitting on my arse reading and writing. During this time, I assumed, some new path would open itself up to me. I secretly hoped it would be a career as a writer, though that was very much a pipe dream.

As it turned out, the academic life suited me rather well, and it became clear that one degree really wasn't enough. Typically, this piece of information had to be pointed out to me, but I was soon knee-deep in Francis Bacon, performing the sort of arcane research which is really an apprenticeship, a way of moving from one world to another.

A few years passed, and around 2005 I began to get itchy fingers. I had almost finished my PhD, my old employers at the magazine asked me to interview a guitar player or two, and I was about to get married. I suddenly realised I missed the grunt and bark of a too-loud electric guitar. So, I dusted down my Strat, re-strung it, gave it a thorough going-over, stuck it in the corner, looked at it, admired it ... waited a few weeks and then finally started to noodle around on it. Nothing too taxing, as I knew my callouses had gone and my fingers would be somewhat rusty, stiff, unresponsive. And so they proved to be. But there was also something else.

When I was at the peak of whatever guitaristic career I possessed, I was what was termed a 'virtuoso'-style player. Though I was far more versatile than most would allow, I was mostly known for my technical aptitude, not least my ability to pick extremely fast and complex single-note lines with, ahem, 'perfect' articulation and accuracy. Basically, I could waggle the fingers on my left hand extremely fast, and pluck each string at exactly the right time for it to reach its full potential as a note. The speed is easy – it's co-ordinating the two hands that's tough.

At first, I tried to persuade myself that it was just ring-rust that was stopping things falling quite into place when I attempted old riffs I used to be able to perform with ease, but I was kidding myself. I simply knew that something else was going on. Something that no amount of practice was going to fix. It strikes me that it must happen something like this for everyone. The symptoms of PD are, unfortunately, quite similar to those of that most common of diseases: getting on a bit. If you take the tremor out of the equation, what you're left with, at least initially, is a couple of symptoms that you might expect anyway at a certain age, namely joint and muscle stiffness and slowly diminishing fine muscle control. Yes, yes, there are bundles of other symptoms, common and not so common, but unless you're particularly sensitive to the ways in which your body works in certain areas, and I mean the areas first affected by PD, you're likely to dismiss the first onset of symptoms with a sigh and a hankering for the lost physical fluidity of youth. And any moaning to others about stiffness, slowness, or a failure to be able to twiddle small things in one hand (PD tends to be quite one-sided, at least at first) is liable to be treated with a knowing glance, a shake of the head and a reminder of your age … and this works from, say, thirty. Sorry everyone, the downhill stretch has already started by then. If you're forty, it's stronger still. Get to the typical age of PD diagnosis, the early sixties, and it needs some special intervention to convince people you're not just getting old, that you're somehow wrong. PD has some special interventions, which is why we're here.

The fact of the matter is, your body changes, and it's only when you feel it oughtn't, when you feel 'wrong', that you even think about doing anything about it. I felt wrong. The karate business had confused me, and the guitar business worried me. So, I decided to investigate.

Making the decision to try to get to the bottom of something that is almost intangible is difficult at the best of times. I found it necessitated just a little bit of untruth – on the assumption that if you over-egg the pudding, make out the possible consequences to be rather more severe than they are, you can get people to move just that little bit quicker. As the problem primarily manifested itself in my left hand, I decided to give the strong impression that I was still a professional guitar player, in order to make the entire thing somewhat more pressing. It worked, to a degree.

My doctor unsurprisingly found nothing wrong at all. He felt – and this still seems to have been utterly reasonable behaviour on his part, even if it was wrong – that the cause was most probably physical, perhaps some sort of trapped nerve. Having suffered from terrible tennis elbow a few years previously from guitar playing, a condition that refused to respond to conventional treatment but was cured almost instantly by a wily physiotherapist, I was perfectly happy with his decision to send me to a physio. Seemed perfectly logical to me.

A month or two of physio not only made no difference, it failed to locate any obvious cause. It may sound ridiculous that a pair of professionals would miss these early signs of PD, but it seems perfectly reasonable to me. Diseases rarely present in straightforward ways, and diagnostics is something of a dark art. My father was a GP (though by this point he was dead, so not a lot of use; it would have been interesting to see what his response would have been, but that's yet another story). He once told me, during the scandal of an undiagnosed case of meningitis at some university or other, that in all his years of doctoring, he'd never seen a single case. And meningitis, for all the publicity, is still pretty rare: in 2009, for example, there were just 1,500 reported cases. For PD, the figures stack up like this: there are 127,000 people in the UK with PD, and one in twenty is diagnosed with what's known as early onset, that is, at age 40 or below. Approximately 10,000 new cases are diagnosed annually, of whom 500 or so will be early onset. To put that into perspective, there are 41,349 GPs in the UK. That means there are over 80 GPs for each of these early onset diagnoses. So a GP of 40 years' practice only has a 50% chance of ever having a patient with early onset PD. Rough figures, but you get my drift. To me, that means it's not the first thing that springs to the average GP's mind when a 40-year-old guitarist says 'my left hand's not working properly'.

So. What did I do next? Well, in traditional fashion, I sort of let it lie. There was no obvious cause, no-one even considered something like PD and my symptoms only seemed excessive to me. Obviously, at this distance, it's difficult to explain why I simply backed off. I knew something was up, even if no-one else could really see it. I knew it wasn't really wear and tear, that it wasn't really down to age, but I sat on it. I bought another guitar, a beautiful handmade flamenco guitar, and I tried another type of playing. New style, new problems, bigger fingerboard, more margin for error ... sometimes I'm quite sneaky, especially with myself. I like to think I'm quite hard to fool, unless it's me doing the fooling. I fall for my own lines every time.

While we might pretend that in hindsight our vision is always 20:20, the past is invariably a lot further away than that. From any reasonable distance it looks really, really small. But I think I just didn't want to know. Subconsciously I understood that the knowledge was going to be something that would change everything. I simply didn't want to know.

They say that a little knowledge is a dangerous thing. Fear of knowledge is even more dangerous. My complacency was soon challenged, however, as my self-imposed stasis turned inexorably into the process of diagnosis.

Creeping like snail unwillingly to school – on diagnosis

Diagnosis is a strange process, and in the case of a disease such as PD, which lacks simple, powerful symptoms, it truly is a process, rather than an instance. The moment at which the process starts is, unlike the first signs, quite easy to pinpoint – and this moment can be quite some time before the first tests are run, the first opinions received. It is from this point that the clock starts ticking. The problem is simply that the clock face is hidden from view. It might be counting down, it might not.

In my case, diagnosis began at a very specific time, and this was not, oddly enough, when I first approached the medical profession with the feeling that something was wrong. My diagnosis began at a party.

Why worry about when the diagnosis begins? I don't know. What I do know is that for me it is indicative of my whole attitude to this disease. It's instructive. It tells me things, some of which I don't really want to know. But them's the breaks. Without getting too poncy about it all, this is a book that demands honesty. It might even get it – I'll cross that bridge when the troll is out. I have struggled with various aspects of this disease, and still do. Not quite having it yet was a struggle, too, but for a very particular set of reasons.

Like I said, my diagnosis began at a party. And it revolved, once more, around my status as a guitar player. No-one in my family or their immediate circle of friends really understood the reasons why I stopped playing the guitar. This is partially because I didn't really understand them myself, and partially because I never volunteered what information I did have. The end result of this lack of comprehension was an incessant flow of well-meaning comments about the music industry, and how I could simply slot back into it again. The chorus reached cacophonic proportions when I finished my PhD and stepped on to the great 'oh, bugger, no-one wants to give me a job' treadmill. Work was scarce, because of what was then called the RAE (Research Assessment Exercise – the process which gives Universities their ranking, and means that they tend only to employ new people who can bring a lot of points with them), because of the economy, because of the time of year … no-one ever said it was because of me, but one does wonder.

The upshot was simple. Every gathering would lead to at least one individual suggesting that it was time to start teaching/playing/writing about the guitar again. For the first few such people, I made an attempt at explaining why, exactly, it was that I wouldn't be playing the guitar again anytime soon. It wasn't complex, though I never quite got into the performance anxiety part of everything, but it seems that well-meaningness quite overwhelms people's ability to listen. Trying to explain always seems mealy-mouthed when the original comment is offered in such good faith. Eventually, I just gave up trying. I went, instead, for the most direct approach – a semi-falsehood allied with a demonstration. Show, don't tell was the order of the day.

I realised that if I tried to waggle my fingers in a sort of digital mexican wave, my right hand was fine, but my left hand, well … it was more than noticeably slower. It juddered, it stalled, it simply failed. The physical demonstration of the indisputable spasticity of my left hand, the one to which falls the task of pressing the strings on to the frets when operating a guitar, succeeded where any amount of reasoned explanation failed. One unimpressive waggle and the subject was all but closed. No great investigation, no enquiries as to why ... it seemed enough to consider that my left hand was simply worn out. After all, every profession takes its toll, sooner or later.

And so on to my mother's 70th birthday party. It was exactly as you would expect, lots of people who hadn't seen me for years, asking for the same update. It's not the first time I've thought I ought to have taken a recent events CV, just to hand out to people before I speak with them. Now my blog takes that role, saving an awful lot of trouble in terms of explanation. But back then there was no blog, no Twitter (for me, at any rate), no real way to explore an individual before you met them. I pretty much started the party waggling my fingers. By the time the party finished I was too drunk to care about finger-waggling, but in the meantime I played out this scenario time after time after time:

They: Why don't you just play the guitar again?

Pete: [to self] Oh god, here we bloody go again ...

They: It just seems ...

Pete: [holding up right hand, waggling fingers furiously] Right hand

They look quizzical. Pete holds up his left hand, waggling his fingers slowly, pathetically.

Pete: Left hand.

They: Oh, I see.

Pete: I just can't do it any more.

They: So, how's the pie? [etc]

At this party, however, things were to take a different turn. Diagnosis was to begin. It strikes me now as odd that while the disease itself entered by stealth, gradually worming its way into my world until I couldn't ignore it any more, my own status changed dramatically three times. It was at this party that change number one happened. I moved from being me to being a potential patient. With the wave of a hand. It truly just happened. One minute I was wafting about the room, talking with people and waggling my fingers like a loon, and the next minute the whole damn process began.

Patient-in-waiting

After one finger-waggling session, I was ushered over by my uncle, a professor of medicine, and I blithely obeyed. Since my father's death my relationship with Michael had changed. No longer did he assume the position of authority, the ultimate family patronage. Now, he treated me almost conspiratorially like an equal. This had confused me momentarily, but was generally most welcome – after all, he's an intelligent, well-respected and distinguished gentleman. Why not indulge in his company? I leant down so that I could hear him speak: 'You need to see a neurologist, old boy.' I may have made up the old boy, and he may have made me do the waggle dance again, but the word neurologist is really all you need to know. It is certainly the word that placed me 'under investigation' ... a patient-in-waiting.

Though this word stung, I was enjoying myself rather, so I nodded my assent and skipped off. Michael rang my mother the next day, telling her to tell me not to forget, and that he was serious – I was under orders. The whole thing was approaching conspiracy theory levels. There were now three in the loop, soon to become four when I told my wife.

You'd think I'd have sprung into action, but it took me six months before I got myself referred to a specialist. This wasn't recalcitrance on the part of my doctor, or sloth on the part of the NHS: this was entirely me.

There are things in life that have a profound effect. One of the most pressing and unpredictable is knowledge. The actual situation you're in and your knowledge thereof are very different things. The reality of your disease doesn't alter ... it simply is. It will do what it will do. The knowledge of it, however, is something very different. It's something that can't be unlearnt. Once you know, you are never the same again. The entire centre of your universe changes, skews, spins, sinks, shifts. And it will never return to where it was. When you know something is wrong, potentially seriously wrong, the fear of walking down an alleyway that admits no turning is palpable. Even allowing for the fact that it is an alleyway down which you must walk.

Annoyingly, by this point one cannot even choose to remain in ignorant bliss. Because you *know*. It's a Rumsfeld, effectively, a known unknown. But it's one that demands discovery.

It was January, 2008 when I found myself walking into a neurologist's lair, putting my coat on the back of the chair, and calmly recounting the story thus far. He poked and prodded, waggled my wrists, made me walk up and down the corridor, made me write stuff, questioned me relentlessly, and poked and prodded me some more.

'So,' he began, 'have you any theories as to what might be going on?'

Now, I'm rarely lost for an answer, and mostly when I appear to be, it's because I have an answer but suspect it might be more politic to keep it to myself. This time, however, I was incapable of transforming my feelings of fear and trepidation into a logical explanation of what exactly it was that ailed me.

'I ask because you're plainly an intelligent man' (I tend to use the appellation 'Dr' whenever I'm in a situation where such things are valued), 'and with your family history' (I had explained that my father and uncle were both doctors), 'I don't think you're liable to freak out'. I paraphrase, naturally, but whatever he said, that's what I heard.

'So I'm going to tell you what I think', he continued, unabated. 'I would be happy to diagnose you with Parkinson's Disease right now, but there are a couple of things which can lead to Parkinsonisms that we're going to test for first.'

This seems to be an appropriate time to explain a few technical things about PD and how it's diagnosed. I'm not going to spend too much time on this because there are plenty of resources available to help you understand what it is (a selection of which I will include at the end of the book), and I'm obviously more interested in the personal, emotional aspects of the disease.

Parkinson's Disease: a short explanation

Parkinson's as a disease is one that falls into the category of 'needs clinical diagnosis', that is, it's not entirely clear when you do have it: there is no 'test', as such, no sure-fire way of diagnosing it, other than the DATSCAN, which detects dopamine deficiency and is fast coming to be considered the final test to confirm diagnosis. Having said that, the process of diagnosis is relatively simple, even if the decision is not. There are things known as Parkinsonisms, which include muscle rigidity (such as cogging, in which the wrists or neck, when moved, feel as if attached to a cogged wheel rather than moving smoothly), akinesia (absence of movement, often appearing as vacant expression, sitting very still), bradykinesia (slowness of movement, often manifest in reduced dexterity) tremor, micrographia (small, often illegible handwriting), problems with walking and balance, a softening of the voice, blah-de-blah ... and these things can be the result of various things, one of which is the lack of dopamine caused by Parkinson's itself. There are tests for dopamine deficiency, specifically the deficiency caused by the death of cells in the section of the brain called the substantia nigra, notably the basal ganglia. A diagnosis of PD depends firstly on the diagnosis of the Parkinsonisms themselves, and secondly the elimination of other possible causes. If it ain't Wilson's (a syndrome caused by an accumulation of copper), or a brain tumour, or one of a handful of other conditions, some eminently curable, some not, then PD is the only thing left.

So. One conversation. Blood tests and an MRI scan to make sure there's not an egg in my head fucking everything up, and we're away. Cool. Great. One sword of Damocles. To go. But confidence rubs off, and the doctor was so confident of his diagnosis that I had no doubt whatsoever that these tests were merely formalities, the confirmation in writing of a deal made with a handshake.

But I didn't *know*. I existed in both a PD/not-PD state simultaneously. A state that contrasted with, that butted heads with, the straightforward nature of the experience. I write like it was perfunctory. Matter-of-fact. That's exactly how it was.

My wife drove me to the station, I got on the train, I opened the *Faerie Queene*, and I glanced through my lecture notes. Allegory and dark conceit. That's what Sir Walter Raleigh talked about in his opening letter. That was the title of my lecture. It's the kind of thing that you expect to hit you, you know, really fucking **HIT** you. That's what happens in the movies, anyway.

Or had she left me to go to work, and I had to get the bus? I don't remember. I felt alone. Utterly.

Did that seem in any way disjointed to you? Well, it's kinda how I felt. Utterly in control and yet entirely divorced from myself. It's something that I have felt since. I explained it once, in a blog post which concentrated on my performance on the cricket field:

Cartesian? Moi? [first published 20 Oct, 2010]

Well, it's quite some time since I wrote anything much, and there are a bundle of reasons for this, some of which may or may not become apparent over the next whatever. Suffice to say it's been an odd and frustrating summer.

It is strange just how much is in one's head, when it comes to doing stuff, and also it is particularly, well, fucking annoying, actually, just how difficult it is to follow one's own prescriptions. In the old days, when I taught guitar to people, some of whom are now proper good (and a few of whom are proper, *proper* good — I had little to do with these ones, I suspect, but hey …) I used to explain to them that during the time in which I was breaking down their old technique and replacing it with a shiny new one, they'd suck for a while, get really frustrated, and wish they'd never bothered. Persevere, I said (quite forcefully, as I'm sure some of them will happily agree). And, well, whaddaya know, I was absolutely right.

So after an off-season spent rebuilding my batting technique, I start to net really well, and enter the season expectant of runs in buckets. Naturally, the cricket gods were watching, and had obviously been to some of my classes back in the day. Why so? Because for the first ten matches or so, if there was a one in twenty chance of getting out, I would. That's what happens when you're out of form. The edge carries, the run-out chance is a direct hit, the overbalancing leads to the ball hitting your big toe and cannoning on to the stumps, the third slip takes an astonishing catch, only to drop a dolly off his own bowling three overs later.

When things aren't going your way, that's the way it stays. And boy, did it stay. I had a short run mid-season, but that was it. My cause wasn't helped by the fact that on taking up a rather more vigorous martial art, I dislocated my shoulder and, well, let's just say things changed.

You see, what I used to tell my students is to relax, let it flow, just let it be. And I used to cheat to make it happen. I'd make them do something so daftly stupidly difficult for them, but really make them try, expecting them to succeed but knowing they'd fail … and when they went back to the original thing, they'd be so disgusted with themselves, or maybe angry, or maybe broken, that … well, it would flow. And once they'd heard it, felt it, caressed it the way it ought to be, that would be it. Barrier broken. Job done. Thank you and goodnight.

But no fucker does this for me, and try as I might, I couldn't make it happen for myself. I once (sorry, Mayfield) got so annoyed after batting myself into the dodgy bowlers only to twat the ball straight up in the air that I put my fist through the pavilion wall. As the opposition captain observed … if only I batted like I punched …

The next, and final game everything changed. Why? Well, because of the Parkinson's (oh, and after two years … count 'em, two … I finally got the genetic results … more on that later) I simply can't jab with my left hand, so when I spar there's an awful lot of dancing about to be done … as I wait until I can actually do something. My defence is vulnerable, so I have had to adapt it. And finally I just relaxed and thought 'fuck it, who cares', and decided I was just not going to get hit. So to speak.

And lo and behold, before I know it, two has turned into ten, ten into twenty … and then I'm being applauded. The opposition keeper has to point out it's because I've just reached my fifty.

Now, this is all well and good, but your point, sir? Hmm … I'm sure I had one … oh yes. Tonight I'm rolling (that is, doing groundwork, wrestling … you know the sort of thing) when my opponent tries something, I try to prevent it, and ker-runch goes my other bloody shoulder.

You see, what I lost during the cricket season, and what I tried so hard to instil in my students, was that flexibility of thought which allows you to take what the world gives you and simply absorb it. Roll with it, so to speak. That's a lesson I finally remembered on that final Sunday of the season. Sadly, my tendons and ligaments aren't following suit. One of the effects of this delightful condition is a loss of the elasticity in said tendons and ligaments … an increased stiffness in the muscles … and when you're working with a partner, and they say 'loosen up', you can only say 'ain't gonna happen' so many times. 'We'll get it', they say. 'Er, no we won't but don't sweat it', I reply. Eventually, I simply tell them.

The point, the point. Well, with Parky's (and no, I have neither the Parkin gene — so odd to have a gene for a kind of ginger bread thing — nor Lrk 2) there are the obvious symptoms — the tremor and the Parkinson's shuffle. Sounds like a dance. And it is, because what's beneath the surface is worse — joints seizing up, loss of fine motor control (hey, look, I have trouble wielding a fork, of course I'm not going to be playing the fucking guitar again), trouble swallowing … er, other stuff I have to look forward to.

Look to what's underneath. Because that's what makes what you can see happen. So much of this life is in the head, and, sometimes, a part of it fucks up, and that, too, affects the outside. My basal ganglia are giving up the ghost. The result is I fall, I get injured, I take longer to heal. My brain is mostly on the money, and then some. But it is communicating less and less well with my body. I am becoming Cartesian. Bugger.

As I sat on that train trundling towards my date with Spenser, I was, as yet, officially undiagnosed. An in-betweenie, stuck between the Scylla of suspicion and the Charybdis of confirmation. I knew that I had PD, but it was as yet unconfirmed. I both did and did not know, I did and did not have it, I could and could not share … this was merely an instance of the fingerpost. This is how my train journey went. Repetition. Unanswerable questions. Repetition.

I was merely midway through the diagnostic process. I recall quite vividly standing at the front of the lecture hall, talking about Spenser as if on autopilot, while my inner voice simply repeated 'I have Parkinson's' over and over, as it tried (in vain), to make some sort of sense of it all. Every so often, in between one of Spenser's delightful lines, it tried to come out, to break out. I wanted to shout it out. As if the burden was too great to bear on my own. Well, it wasn't the burden at all. Nothing so prosaic. It wasn't trying to come out, to break out, to shout out … it was more like a rather delayed response to it all. More of an 'I'm sorry, did I hear that right? Parkinson's, did you say?' It is a commonplace that as you stand and lecture, you feel fraudulent. You feel as if you have no real knowledge of what you teach, as if your students are sitting, laughing at you and your ignorance behind their notepads and frayed school-vintage pencil cases. You shouldn't be teaching, you're still a student yourself. Ezra Pound suggested that the best teachers acted as if they were discovering the material along with their students. This state of unknowing is very similar to the mid-diagnostic state. It's your own body, it's telling you something important, but in a code neither you nor anyone else has cracked.

I lectured, I took seminars, I stayed where I always stayed in London when lecturing … then lectured again, took more seminars. Went home. Beyond that, it's all a bit of a blur. I may even have made some of it up, invented feelings I didn't have to make up for my not having had them. When I got home, what happened? You know, I have no idea. My wife and I talked, … well, we must have done. But the timing was simply awful. It couldn't have been worse if it'd been scripted. We were, at this point, in the final stages of IVF. This, for those of you lucky enough not to have experienced it, is quite astonishingly stressful. For various reasons, our experience was perhaps even more stressful than most. And then this. We polarised. We fell apart. Gently. Carefully. Unobtrusively. Irrevocably.

We still went to Zanzibar over the summer, where I practised karate on the beach every morning at five, and we had one of the more surreal holidays imaginable. By the September of that year I had left the marital home. By November we had sold up. It was a sad end to what had been five mostly very good years, but I'm lurching ahead. This was merely one of the trajectories that life had in store for me. I was still officially undiagnosed. Now it was time to wait until I received the letter that contained the appointment that contained the test that would deliver the verdict. It was perhaps indicative of the state of our relationship that this next stage was something I experienced entirely alone. It was time for the MRI.

The day of my scan was a very strange one. I attended the clinic alone (it may have been by choice ... I honestly cannot remember the reason), I drove to the hospital – almost forty-five minutes away – and parked my car. Naturally, I parked far, far away from the neurology department. But eventually I found my bearings, signed in and was ushered to the waiting room. So, I've been semi-diagnosed with a rather tedious disease and I'm feeling rather alone and, strangely, a little bit scared. This is not the time for confrontation. This is not the time to be sat beside one's own fragility, with the ghosts of my future, like some latter-day Scrooge.

This is why I question the wisdom of having a waiting room in the lounge of one of the wards. I'm possibly very ill. I don't know yet. I'm here to find out. Sorry, but what I don't want is to be sat in a ward full of people with serious neurological problems, wondering quietly to myself which one is me, and when. It was impossible not to notice that certain patients were in the advanced states of cerebral decay. At one point a patient shuffled into the waiting area, where I sat in a high-backed 70s armchair looking at the pile of women's magazines trying to work out why there are never any men's magazines. Not that I would read them anyway. She shuffled in and began talking to me as if she and I had known each other for years. I think she mistook me for a member of her family. Oddly enough, though the basic response to this situation was fear, fear of what I might become, in many ways it completely divorced me from my self. I had become many ... well, perhaps just two. There was me as me, and me as patient. I didn't want to be a patient.

I waited.

Eventually, a nurse fluttered into the ward and ushered me towards the place where they keep the MRI machine, a different department down the usual long corridors and past big important signs and all the other stuff that you fixate upon when on an unknown route. My ball of twine was writ in black and white and blue and yellow. But of course, I really just followed the arrows.

The machine is kept in a far more organised space than the ward, but also one more brutal. This is the machine that slices and dices you, that gives you pictures of sections of your brain. It has a reputation, claustrophobics hate them, apparently – the operator gives you a panic button. In its presence there are no secrets, so you immediately divest yourself of your clothing and don a delightful hospital gown. Then you're called in.

The machine itself is a big lump with a tube into which the patient is inserted. It's quite snug. I can see why people freak out, the combination of fear of what it'll find and its malevolent air is quite powerful. One of the intimidating things about the scanner is that it needs you to remain perfectly still for the 25-30 minutes for which it assaults your senses, with no recourse available. There is simply nowhere to go.

Still. Perfectly still. (Incidentally, I picked up the DVD of my head on March 15th. Beware the ides of March indeed. Like Julius Caesar, I was done in by those closest to me, my own brain cells.) The stillness is not optional. It's no use having twenty minutes of scan and then going blurry. There are, naturally, ways and means of keeping various parts of your body still. For the head, it's a headcase. Quite literally. A clear perspex case into which your head fits, making you feel like a badly paid extra playing a badly made alien in Doctor Who. I lay on my back, and was slid gently into the machine. Above my face was a mirror at 45°, presumably to ensure that I remained connected to the outside world. Without my glasses, though, all I could see were a pair of blurry feet and the form of the radiologist as he had a sip of his coffee before asking me if I was comfortable in my coffin. He didn't call it my coffin, of course, but the top of the patient-hole is remarkably low. With my hands on my chest I could have touched it simply by flexing my wrists.

The MRI machine takes photographs of slices of your head, like the delightful one on the next page, and it seems to do that by trying to drill a hole in your skull through simple bone-crushing volume. This machine is loud, quite astonishingly loud. I've stood next to drummers and bass players who pride themselves on the sheer mass of their sonic attack, and yet would skulk away, embarrassed at their sheer wimpiness when confronted with this beast. It also hurls a quite breathtaking variety of sounds at your body – the volume is of the sort that doesn't bother itself with your ears, but goes straight for the spinal column. It's a pneumatic drill, then a drum kit, then a hydraulic ram, then a generator, then a train ... and it goes on and on and bloody on ... and then goes on some more.

After something approaching half an hour of this cruel and unusual punishment, the disorientation sets in with a vengeance. It's more existential than physical, a bone-deep confusion. It's a little like one of those mornings when you wake and have no real idea of where you are, or who you are, and there's that slightest suspicion that it might just be because you truly don't know where or who you are.

I have a sneaking suspicion that I fell asleep.

I was dragged out of the machine and sent on my way, conscious that now the scans needed to be interpreted before anyone could make any decision.

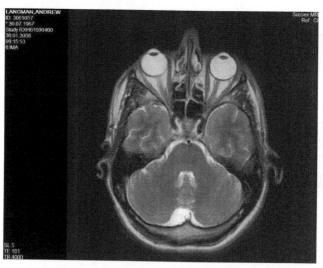

This is my brain. Oh, and my eyes, and nose ...

The status of my patienthood was soon to become clear. But not before I had waited for another hour or two. So I waited.

It's odd how waiting rooms are so monumentally unfit for purpose. Either that or those occupying them are monumentally unfit for the task at hand. It's easier to wait in the machine, to be honest. More relaxing, too. I suppose this is because there's consistency enough for the brain to switch off, and too much stimulation to get bored. After what seemed like some time, yet another consultant trooped in and led me away. This time, it was for 'the talk'. This was the part of the day that would define my future. From this moment on … well, some upcoming moment, anyway.

It may be pertinent to consider the gravity of the situation here. I don't mean in terms of illness, because if anything, the moment of official diagnosis marks a point of improving health, as from then on we, the patient, can be given drugs and therapies, put on programmes, enrolled in support groups. The illness, the dysfunction, the physiological cock-up, these will continue in their own sweet, oblivious manner, without giving even the tiniest of tosses about l'il ole us. But diagnosis has a whole host of implications, carries with it a great truckload of neuroses, is accompanied by great swathes of symptoms. In short, diagnosis means that *we* can be put in a very specific box. The box marked thus:

PATIENT

[PD]

Patronise completely.

Nowhere to put the waiting room? No worries, we'll just stick it in a ward. Simple. Short on consultation rooms? No problem. We'll just borrow this patient's room while he/she is off having lord knows what done to him/her.

It's a very strange feeling sitting in a long-term patient's room. The walls are covered in posters, charts, action plans, photographs, as if their memory is the thing that's broken so they have to pin it up. Of course, this may well be the case. You feel as if you're trespassing inside someone else's life, and this, of course, is because you are. When you're expecting the worst, the last thing you want to do is feel like you're intruding on someone else's illness.

My consultant is young, and British Asian. These facts are entirely irrelevant, but they are facts. She begins to talk about the scans, explaining that nothing abnormal is showing up, and there's nothing going on in the various blood tests. The genetic tests are yet to return, because they often take in excess of three months (I think in my case it was over 30), and while I forget the exact phrase she used, it was something along the lines of 'for us, no news is bad news'. That is, the original diagnosis has yet to be contradicted, nullified, by a slew of 'other factors'.

This part of proceedings is very stressful. I try, but I find it hard to hold on to, process, and listen to everything she has to say. And it's not just me who's finding things stressful, as she, too, seems a little nervous. This doesn't much surprise me, but I'm not sympathetic, even though I really ought to be. She begins to run through the various treatments in use, describing the ways in which the dopamine deficiency might be tackled. She suggests that we start off on a low dose of a dopamine agonist, that is, a drug that aims to give those naughty basal ganglia a kick in the pants, and convince the ones still alive to up their game in the dopamine production stakes. We're going to start with a low dose of pramipexole, branded as Mirapexin, which should begin to bring my recalcitrant left hand back into the game.

'Hang on ...' I interrupt her mid-flow, 'are you telling me I've definitely got Parkinson's?'

'Oh', she replies, 'didn't I say that?'

She looked a little stunned, and not a little embarrassed. Now, I know that the answer's yes, but ... well, diagnosis is not complete without those words being heard, is it?

'No', I say.

There is a short silence, before she simply states that yes, I do have PD.

These few words change everything.

I am now a PWP (though I didn't learn this abbreviation for another three years). I am now a patient. I am now no longer simply me. I am one of few, a select group to which no-one wishes to belong.

I am now a patient.

Perhaps asking that question was a strategy on my part. A strategy to force me to confront the illness, and one that forced her to be the most uncomfortable person in the room. On the other hand, I may merely have wanted to know what I already knew, to hear someone else say the words.

The rest of the session flies by in a blur. I ask the usual questions. What's the prognosis? What next? What should I do? The answer to them all is a simple 'don't know'. Parkinson's is a funny disease. Its diagnosis is clinical (as I mentioned, a matter of elimination of other possible sympomatic causes) and while it's progressive and degenerative, within the general downward trend you can go up and down like a yo-yo.

'Would you mind if some students came in to prod you around a bit?' she asks.

My day can't get any more surreal, can it? I agree. Plus I am well aware that without patients allowing students to prod and poke them, the students won't turn into doctors who know what's what.

Well. Luckily, I was right. But the five medics on a neurology course can barely hide their embarrassment when confronted by a fit, young, articulate individual whose brain just happens to be gently misfiring. I run through the whole story as they try to work out what's wrong, how they would find out, and what tests they might order. To me it's now mundane. The balance of power swings once more.

After several hours I escape clutching a small bag of drugs and get back into my car and drive home. Radio 4 is on, as ever. They advertise a Panorama special, on the hidden side-effects of some drug therapies that, they say, have ruined lives. My life has just changed irrevocably thanks to the labelling of a set of symptoms as caused by something that, if not treatable, is at least open to some measure of symptomatic relief. The last thing I want to hear is that the exact drugs sitting on the passenger seat next to me, shuffling slightly in their white paper bag like so many mice could cause, among other things, compulsive gambling.

Now, you would have thought that was that, but no. There's more, there's always more. With progressive conditions, diagnosis is progressive, too. Quiet time becomes a time to diagnose new symptoms, new indications. New things are immediately smothered with suspicion.

I have yet to gamble away my house.

With a woeful ballad –
on telling people

And as if all of that wasn't enough, as if you weren't simply overwhelmed with the enormity of it all, as if you weren't struggling to make sense of this, this thing, this label you woke up to on your bedside table, there's everybody else. The straightforward if mildly circumlocutory manner in which my various consultants chose to make me aware of my new status as patient began to make a little more sense. It's as if, once diagnosis was confirmed, patient and doctor now began to workshop the dissemination of this information. So, small rather confused person. How does this make you feel? Well, just remember that you can't walk away.

No-one really runs workshops explaining how to tell people you've become a patient, that your world now revolves around the failure of an obscure group of cells in your head to bloody well get on with it, to stop being such divas and bloody well make some more dopamine. Throughout the whole process of diagnosis there's an expectation of some sort of closure. The cause of the strangenesses will be discovered and, well, that will be that. Medicine will be provided, and we can all get back to beetroot farming or whatever it is we do. Safe in the knowledge. The knowledge safe with us.

But there are three words that mean this simply won't wash. Progressive. Degenerative. Incurable. They change the game. Life will never be the same, and yet … and yet you can lay money on the fact that no-one will know that you are having real problems, let alone that you are seeking answers. .

The first person you tell will be one of the very few aware of what's been going on, so they will have been as primed as you are. They'll probably know next to nothing about the disease, but then it's highly likely that you're in the same position.

I am the kind of person who finds things out. When PD entered into the event horizon, I did what I usually do: research. Unusually, it didn't work. My eyes sucked in the words and simply funnelled them directly into the trash bin. It was as if knowing more about it would make it all the more inevitable, make it my fault. Immediately after diagnosis I was too busy being busy to think much about it. It was, and so what was the point? Other people, however, have different ideas.

The irony is that of all the chapters here, this one is proving the most difficult. How do I tell thee? Let me count the ways This may well be because I am still telling people. But then, if this is the case, you'd think I'd pretty much have it down by now, right? Well, here's the rub. I actually feel guilty.

The great telling goes pretty much in a spiral, with those closest to you being the first ones to find out. So far, so obvious. This is also something of a mixed blessing. It is in some ways a very good thing, as they invariably know something's up, and when the time comes for the conversation, they can pretty much tell what it's going to be about. It's a little like when you sit your partner down and explain to them that it's not working out, it's time to move on, the spark has gone, however you describe it. They see you coming. And this is when the rather unexpected guilt started – for me, at any rate.

So. I'm sitting trying to write about success, about the roles we assume, and have thrust upon us, without much luck. Why? Well, the point I am trying to make is simple. It's just that I'm failing to make it simple. We all assume roles within our various relationships, and these roles are based, more or less, on our own view of success and what it means. I am one of those people who can set myself a target and yet, when (or if) I hit it, will happily put it down to its lack of ambition, or explain it away in terms that devalue it. If I can achieve it, where's the achievement? In many ways, my life has been one in which I set goals, achieve them, and then deny the achievement. What is success? Twitter came to my rescue this morning:

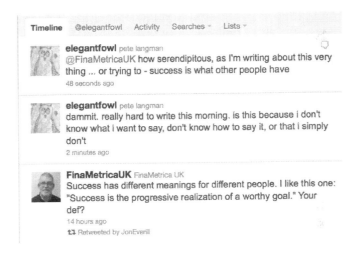

Which I thought was very kind of it, all in all. The definition proffered here is perhaps more astute than it realises. Ignoring the word 'worthy', for perhaps obvious reasons, we are left with two points that are somewhat at odds: 'progressive realisation' and 'goal'. I suspect (though I may be wrong), that the writer intends the goal to be the measure of success – after all, a goal is either achieved or not achieved. But the achievement itself leads to an empty, goal-less state that must be filled with a new goal. This can be problematic (it certainly is for me). The idea of progressive realisation, however, is far more interesting. In these terms the goal itself is not the achievement, as the real success lies in the knowledge that one is gradually moving towards it. This movement as success promotes continuous feelings of belonging, unthreatened by the irritation of having to refocus on a new, more difficult to achieve goal.

My formulation, 'success is what other people have', is far more cynical. And yet it was what I was brought up to believe.

Now comes a really difficult decision. Do I tell you, and if so, how? How will you react? What will you say? What will you do? Will you walk away?

It'sa bit like when I tell people I really never got on with my father. On his deathbed he confided in me: 'I never understood why we didn't get on.' Possibly the dumbest thing he ever said. I contemplated explaining it to him, but chose the better part of valour. Which made a change. When it came to me, he rarely did. It's a dull father/son story that everyone has heard a thousand times before, and it's immeasurably duller for failing to involve any physical abuse of any kind. A few quotations should do.

On gaining A level English
'But you can't even speak the language.'

On deciding to become a musician:
'I can understand your sister wishing to do this: she's got talent'

On postgraduate studies
'You know we all think it's a complete waste of time'

On marriage (said to my future mother-in-law)
'He won't make her happy'

For the record, he was a very fine doctor, from what I understand, even if he had a love/hate relationship with the profession. But we didn't get on.

So. Perhaps that's not much of a secret, perhaps it's nothing much to write home about, perhaps you don't really care. The fact is, I know how people react to this 'revelation', I just can't always pin the reaction to the person. And so it was when I began to tell people about my diagnosis, when I began to tell them about the PD. To them, it was one negotiation. To me, it's a continuous process, surprising at every turn. Sometimes good, sometimes bad. I've been telling people for four years now, and will continue to do so. To all of you I've told, my apologies. To all of you I have yet to tell, my apologies.

The problem is that people react in such completely different ways, and you can never tell who will react how. In the beginning, I mostly told people in concert with my wife. It was 'our news'. This, naturally, posed some difficulties. We struggled on occasion to pick the right moment, waiting until we were far too drunk to have a coherent discussion on the subject. Looking back, I think this may have been a very good approach, if only because it freed us from having to answer various awkward questions. The tension in the air is also palpable when you're searching for the 'right moment'. It doesn't help when one of you says the immortal words 'we've got something to tell you': code the world over for 'we're having a baby'. Cue really uncomfortable reactions. Disappointment is a strange reaction to observe in another when you tell them you've somehow acquired a progressive, degenerative, incurable brain disease.

The reactions. Now there's an interesting study. No two have been the same, because no two people are the same. All the same, I'm going to put together some basic categories, just to make things easier for me.

Guilt (theirs)

This is mostly reserved for parents and relations who assume that they have passed the disease on. This may be true, though the genetic markers for PD do not inevitably lead to the disease, nor does having ancestors who suffered with it automatically lead to you developing it. It is fair to say that they increase the likelihood of your developing it, however. This feeling is often accompanied by the desire that they, not you, had developed it, by statements that it isn't fair, and so on. The very few times I've come across this, I've ended up being the one dispensing solace and advice. This is plainly nuts, but just as the initial instinct is to look backwards in a vain attempt to see exactly where things started to change, the family scour their collective memories to find the link: the person who had it before. My mother did this, and decided that her grandmother may have had PD, but as she died when my mother was six, it was impossible to say for sure. Plainly, it was simply impossible. This didn't deter her from fretting about something she couldn't change even if she knew for sure. I'm not surprised at her reaction, nor do I in any way wish to criticise it. But I certainly wasn't expecting it. In addition to those who assume guilt for your disease, there are also those who seem to consume it, as if it were theirs alone. They are rare, but I've met a couple. Frankly, they freaked me out.

Guilt (yours)

There have been several times when I've felt guilty when sharing the news. Telling partners and children is particularly fraught. Even though my wife knew about the problems, knew about the initial diagnosis, knew about the MRI scan, knew when she would know, I was still aware that those few words changed everything. Naturally, I can't answer for her, nor would I try to, but there were things in my relating the positive diagnosis that were inescapable, and for which I felt monumentally guilty. I had been reticent enough on the subject of children beforehand, but now I simply couldn't envisage our having any.

The first issue was the possibility of passing on the disease, even though this was not a given, nor one with any statistically designated likelihood. And that's ignoring the possibility of medical advances in treatment that may have obtained in the next forty years. Stem cell research is highly unlikely to come to my aid, if only because of the time it takes to license a treatment, especially one so controversial, but there's no reason why it might not be successful in forty years or so. Probably much, much earlier.

The second, and to me more pressing, issue, was that of fatherhood. How could I be the father I never had if I were barely able to walk? If I shook continually, dribbled when I ate, mumbled when I spoke? I simply could not bear the thought of my children being embarrassed by their father, looking at me with pity. Having to look after me.

This little problem, that of my future incapacity, also made me feel guilty when telling her. It felt a bit like telling her that I was a fraud, not the man she thought she was marrying but a shop-soiled version, one that ought to have been recalled to the factory, replaced with a new model of equal or greater value. Oh, by the way, the physically fit man you married? Broken. Soon you'll be mopping up after him. This may seem extreme, and in many ways it was, but I had tunnel vision. All I could see was the 'goal', and not the process.

As for telling my daughter? Kayleigh, I'm sorry for how it came out. I do wish I had been able to tell you the 'right' way. I wish I had known a 'right' way to tell you. The right way to tell you. But some things simply are.

Telling new or potential partners is also hugely problematic. I might save that until later.

Embarrassment

Quite often I find people squirming with what I can only assume is embarrassment. It seems to be a function of cognitive dissonance – that is, they really want to be nosey and ask loads of questions, but feel that this might be construed as ghoulish. Oddly, I think the person they're most worried about is themselves, as they fear that they'll become one of the things they loathe, like a dyed in the wool thesp suddenly developing a penchant for Big Brother: all the intellectualising in the world won't wash away the faint taste of bile that rises into the back of the throat as they realise who they've become. I have had innumerable conversations with people on the subject of PD, having just informed them of my 'status', in which, after three or four minutes, they ask the same question: 'you don't mind talking about it, do you?' The only logical answer, and the one I always give, is 'obviously not, or I would have changed the subject by now'.

'You don't mind …' is not a question for you, it's a question for them, and it really means 'can you please work on the assumption that this whole conversation is about you, and not about my personal greed for information?' I'm not complaining, nor am I criticising their approach, as it makes perfect sense. To a degree, we are all taken aback when discovering something unexpected, especially when it has a reputation, or is surprising. It is up to the sufferer, or whatever you like to call the person with the disease, to put the other at their ease. It's easy to forget the shock such a piece of information causes in the unprepared. It didn't take long before to me the information was commonplace, mundane even. The person you tell is told once, and once only, whereas each telling is for you a dilution of the shock of the new. Each reaction can seem stranger as a result: you're cool with it, so why the big issue?

Many years ago, I was teaching at a music school in London, and left my tuner there after a class. The composition tutor, who knew I was gigging that evening and that a tuner was a useful addition to my armoury, took it home with him as he lived close by, and gave me a call. I trotted over to pick it up. He answered the door and I made to shake his hand, but stopped before my arm really moved. He spotted it. It was automatic. He was a trombonist who had suffered the effects of his mother being prescribed thalidomide when he was in her womb. I knew this, because I knew him, though not well. But I was mortified. He said nothing, and invited me in. In his living room, he moved to his case, one of those boxy, pilot's cases, flipped off the two lids, pulled my tuner out, spun it up into the air, caught it, and handed it to me. Smiling. He knew I'd freaked myself out, and he knew how to make it cool.

If it's starting to sound like a process, then that's exactly how it feels. The continuous and ever-evolving technique of informing people that you are a PWP is, in effect, a continuation of diagnosis. Indeed, it often feels like you're back with one of the many doctors and consultants and nurses and whoever as you answer the same list of questions, and the same reactions, the same silences, the same embarrassed pauses, the same look in the eyes. These days, I have to concentrate hard not to roll my eyes and drum my fingers on the counter as I switch on the autopilot and let my mouth react to the same old stimuli. I have to remind myself that while I might have heard these same questions over and over again, this is the first time that this individual has asked them. The conversation usually goes something like this.

Me: Actually, there's a reason for 'x', as I have Parkinson's Disease.
They: [pausing] Oh. [another pause] You wouldn't know it ...
Me: Well, there are drug therapies, and there's more to it than the tremor.
They: You're very young.
Me: Well, it's early, yes. One in twenty are diagnosed before they are past 40.
They: My Gran/Uncle/mate's dad ... I think they had it. But they were old.
Me: Yes. It more usually develops in the early sixties.
They: [pause] Didn't that actor have it?
Me: Michael J Fox, yes. He still does.
They: I thought so.

And so it continues. At some point they will get to the questions you can't answer, not least 'what's the prognosis?' This is always awkward. Because you don't know. And, quite naturally, the whole disease is under control just so long as you are able to answer all the various questions hurled in your general direction. At the moment the answer involves a pause, and the words 'now that's a good question', then suddenly everything's out of control. And then it gets awkward again.

This scenario will play out and out and out and out, with the only difference being how obvious it is that there's something wrong. I've started to have people say, 'I wondered why ...' rather than 'you wouldn't know'. There will come a time when I won't need to tell anyone. It will be obvious. I can already see it in others. Seeing it in others, of course, is a particularly affecting experience, and one giving rise to two particular emotional responses. The first is empathy, of course, as you know, really *know*, what it is they're feeling in quite a specific sense. The second is fear, as you see not only how other people see you, but what you will become. This blog post was originally written in response to a piece by Zoe Williams in which she suggested that civilised behaviour vanishes in those few shopping days before Christmas.

It never reins [first published 25 Dec, 2010]

Shopping on Christmas ante-eve is, frankly, a heart-breakingly stupid thing to attempt. There are several problems with it (though, note well Ms Williams, no-one to my knowledge dispensed with all pretence of civilisation ...), all of which are accentuated by the plain simple fact that at such times these shops operate well above capacity. The aisles are designed for about half the number walking round hoovering up goods like the apocalypse is coming. This in itself is a right royal pain, but the constant hoovering means constant re-stocking, turning the normally free-flowing aisles into a microcosmic M25 in the snow.

But this is not very exciting, or even interesting. I buy lots of stuff, and have a discussion regarding the pronunciation of paprika. Is it papp-reeka, or is it papree-ka? This is hardly high-end stuff.

So. A trolley stuffed full of stuff, I park and carefully load it onto the conveyor belt, keen to make my packing as efficient as possible, and to take up as little space as possible. On doing this, I notice the couple to my right … late 50s/early 60s, and note in him the faintest tremor. As I may have mentioned before, I want to reach out (metaphorically speaking) … but I don't. One reason is that just after I notice, and I start processing, my careful packing encounters a design flaw on the check-out. Where the 'next person' shopping dividers are kept all slidily convenient, they encroach upon the belt. The belt advances, the dividers remain aloof. The shopping accommodates.

It does rather more than accommodate, however, as one of the bottles of wine simply makes way, leaping suicidally onto the floor, where it bursts spectacularly at my fellow-shopper's feet.

I'm sure Ms Williams would have assaulted me with her celery, or something, for daring to invade her tiny, super-important, ever-so-amazing world … luckily, the real world is populated with people who have real problems, and for whom life truly is too short to worry about such things. I think Sainsbury's paid to have his jeans dry-cleaned. And that was that.

I hit my head on the bottom corner of a kitchen cabinet door while loading the fridge. That's how thrilling a day I had.

But I take perverse pleasure in these
interactions. As Lear would have said while
waiting for the Gloucesters to visit for
dinner: let me clean the kitchen. It smells
of … mortality.

This is how awareness goes. The continual telling is a
diagnosis in itself, with the symptoms getting progressively
worse, the explanation progressively less shocking, the
reaction less marked. The prognosis less distant.

When I was first diagnosed, telling people was hard, as it felt
like quite an aggressive act, partially because of the reactions
it engendered. My symptoms are now worse with drug therapy
than they were without it when I was first diagnosed, so I can
only guess at what I would be like without the drugs. You still
need to be pretty astute to really notice that something is
wrong. You need to spot how I hold my fork, how I develop a
tiny tremor at certain points, how my left foot shuffles rather
than walks, and I hide these defects well. But there are times
when it is simply necessary to tell someone. I've always been
wary of being defined by this disease, even though I write
about it relentlessly, and to this end it's not something I
introduce into a conversation until it's necessary – this also
avoids causing discomfort in the other until I really need to.
But I have discovered several points when disclosure becomes
inevitable, necessary.

Sports

When training or playing sports, there are times when the PD
simply intervenes. When I was a practising martial artist (and I
never was particularly good, just keen and diligent), I would
often get partners starting to tell me to do 'x' more with my

left-hand when sparring. 'That's not going to happen, I'm afraid,' is my usual answer. Sometimes I add 'trust me' on the end. Sometimes it works. At other times their well-meaning advice boxes me into a corner. 'Oh, we can get the jab/grip/combination of hand-holds working soon enough.' No matter that my left arm simply refuses to jab, or to grip a cricket bat properly, or to be capable of supporting my bodyweight from two of its fingers. It can definitely be sorted out. After two or three rounds of this 'we can sort it' / 'no we can't' I stop proceedings and say 'it won't happen, because I have PD, and my left arm is rather beleaguered, to say the least'. Then we're back to 'the conversation'. One of my less endearing qualities is my ability to become more and more frustrated with some particular action, one that I know is unlikely to occur with any great skill, until I cannot stand it any more. This irritates and upsets me and worries and confuses those around me, even those who know. As time continues apace, this behaviour has diminished, and this is simply because I have developed a far deeper instinctive understanding of what PD means to me.

Possibly the greatest hindrance to contentment is the frankly cretinous idea that to achieve something one merely has to work hard. This is delusional rubbish, and seems to lead an awful lot of people down roads that can only lead to ever more spectacular and public humiliation. I have no problem with ambition, and know full well that without dedication and hard work nothing is ever going to happen, but failure of the type that is inevitable is damaging. What PD has quite merrily demonstrated to me is that of all the judgements one can make, that of self-assessment trumps them all. The ability, and willingness, to work out what is feasible and what is not is worth gold. Yes, you may still fail, but failure at something within one's grasp, while frustrating, is simply life. Failure to achieve something well beyond you is different: the attempt itself is simply embarrassing.

In sports, I have become quite adept at working out what is and is not possible. I know my left side is compromised, so I train to accommodate that, in all sports. I don't attempt holds that require my left-hand fingers alone to support my weight: they will fail. I don't try to penetrate an individual's defences with my left hand: it will fail. Awareness of my weaknesses allows me to succeed, because it allows me to aim for things at which I can succeed. This is perhaps obvious, and obtains in any situation, but for me, PD has accentuated this negotiation between the world and my body.

It can also lead to radical decisions, like my decision to bat left-handed in the 2012 cricket season. This I have calculated as being within my grasp. Time will tell as to whether I'm right, and whether I work hard enough and intelligently enough (since I wrote this, 2012 has been and gone, and I did OK, though perhaps not as well as I'd have liked ... plus ça change).

New relationships

Like many of us in these strange, strange days, I have embraced the internet as a way of meeting new people. It began when my ex-wife and I split and I realised that I knew virtually no-one in my adopted home who wasn't of 'our circle'. This was simply because I'd moved from London to live with her, and everyone I met was either a new friend to us both, or one of her existing circle. This made meeting new people necessary, both to assert my own independence and for rather more salacious purposes. There was a point when my dating behaviour spiralled out of control somewhat, and I was rather over-zealous in finding new friends, and let's be honest here, new lovers. That's for another chapter, but one constant, with every single individual I met, was that they didn't know that I suffered from PD.

The internet, in the form of social media and especially dating websites, allows for an extreme version of the games we play out in pubs and at parties. It allows one to re-invent oneself at will. A new photograph, a witty line, a white lie or two; all these recreate the I, and to some extent literally. This isn't Walter Mitty time, but how we behave in the real world is influenced by how we project ourselves in the virtual. Except that this distinction is quite invalid.

I have met a lot of women online. The question is, when do I broach the subject of PD? When does one slip it into a conversation with a potential lover, partner? Experience tells me that telling before a physical meet often leads to one response ... 'er, don't take this the wrong way ...' I have not met with some potentially lovely people because of this. If you're reading me now, you're probably thinking 'wow, lucky escape', and you may be right.

My blog is quite concerned with PD, so having not told someone online that I am a PWP, my next judgement is always whether to give out my real name. After all, no-one meets someone without googling them these days.

Mostly, I tell when it looks like we'll meet again. And even that makes me feel like a fraud, as if I've met under false pretences. It's the bit where I get embarrassed, slightly lost for words, and vulnerable. It's really not a surprise that sometimes I'm accused (though not vehemently) of exploiting my disease for my own gratification. This has probably been true on occasion, though one ought not underestimate the power of a disease that will cause trouble one day for bringing out the nurturing instincts. But this is allied with a feeling that if the telling is to be done, 'tis best done quickly.

I have terminated several relationships, whether wittingly or unwittingly, because I feel that making a commitment is in some ways insane, because there will come a point when I become dependent. When I truly am 'not the man I first met …' but then, who is?

Perhaps the most interesting 'tell' is when you realise that the person you're telling also has something they wish to share. This is so powerful that the relief can be overwhelming, and overwhelmingly physical.

Over the past four years, I have developed a way and time of disclosing. I tell when it's necessary; never before. And I simply tell it straight.

I have Parkinson's Disease.

Would you like another drink?

Seeking the bubble reputation –
on deciding what it means

So. You've noticed strange stuff afoot. You sweated through the process of diagnosis, and had patienthood thrust upon you. You've tackled the rather unsettling business of telling people. You've found that people have a rather annoying habit of asking you questions. They ask questions like 'what does it mean?' This is quite the most irritating question possible, of course, not least because it's so astoundingly open-ended. This, of course, is why they ask it. It covers practically everything while seeming utterly vague and yet suitably comforting. Within this one question lurks all those things they want to ask but don't dare; those answers they want to hear but don't know are waiting for them. It is the perfect question.

What they don't realise is that when the diagnosis came, it meant everything and nothing, and you had no idea which way to turn. You probably found yourself sitting on the wreckage of your perceived good health, intoning the word 'fuck' repeatedly, interspersed with the odd 'why me?' before returning to 'fuck'. Well, that's what I did anyway. How the bloody hell do I know what it means? This is what my head screams while my lips quietly intone the words, 'well, that's a very interesting question'.

The fact is that while diagnosis may have provided one small answer, what it really did was to usher in the great flood of questions that accompany a progressive, degenerative disease. The questions are continuous, new, and varied. You and your condition are on a mutual voyage of discovery, and it's not entirely clear who's leading the way. More questions than answers.

Most people know about Parkinson's. It has a reputation. It is the disease of age and infirmity. This is where most people's knowledge ends. They may have an inkling that it's a disease that causes the sufferer gradually to lose control of their body, while the mind mostly stays there or thereabouts, but probably not. Yes, there are psychological problems that obtain with PD – after all, your brain has sort of broken, and this isn't going to happen entirely without some sort of knock-on effect – but primarily it is the disease that makes you shuffle, mumble, drool and *shake*. They almost certainly won't know that 5% are diagnosed on or before the age of 40. I am part of that 5%, a few years down the line. They'll probably know the shaking bit, though. This question will always be on the tip of their tongue. That is, why aren't you shaking? If you have already developed a tremor, then it all makes more sense to them.

So, what does it all mean? The answer to the question has many parts. One is 'not what you think'. Another is to list the various symptoms.

How do you affect me? Let me count the ways.

PD is at heart a movement disorder (though this view is currently being challenged by some). Primarily, it does stuff to the way that your muscles behave, by messing up the system by which you order them about. This we know full well. It affects the way you walk. The way you talk. The way you move, the way you shake. The way you eat, the way you drink. The way you piss. Is this what it means?

It will change the way you live. Is this what it means?

It changes the way you see things. Is this what it means?

What it means depends not on the disease, but on you. This

is because its meaning is a product of the questions you ask of it. That and the way in which you decide to treat its answers. PD asks questions continually. Each time it asks, I discover something new about it, and I learn something new about me.

But I'm never prepared for those times when I stop being able to feel. And there have been a few. Here's a blog post which I wrote after one such incident that I still remember quite clearly.

Never quite so alone [first published 29 Sept, 2011]

One never quite feels loneliness as the visceral force it can be as one does when in the close company of others, when one's actions dictate another's; when you cannot lead, no-one can follow.

Recently I began to learn how to tango. It is a dance of detached intimacy, one which invites the closeness of sexual union while simultaneously keeping the partners at one remove — when the man's leg goes forward, the woman's retreats. The word tango comes directly from the Latin tangere, to touch — it is the first person singular. I touch. And yet it takes two, both literally and anecdotally. A dance of contradictions. She wore a plate around her neck: noli me tangere, for Caesar's I am. A dance of eternal chase, a Zeno's paradoxidance.

Noli me tangere. Jesus, too, used these words. Don't touch me.

And I have some natural flair. But the disease, oh this fucking disease. It disconnects. It disconnects you from yourself, from everyone you love, from everything that you've ever chosen as self-definition. It takes it all, and it fucks it. And then some.

One of the many, many irritating little things it does is fuck up your gait. It takes the way you walk and rips the piss. I went to a military academy for six months. There I marched, a habit yet to leave me. Except my left foot is beginning to shuffle. Thud, scuff, thud, scuff.

The tango is fundamentally a poncy walk, done in time to rather groovy music. I can do rhythm. Really.

Tonight, however, is different. From the very first dance, I feel my partner is stiff, unresponsive — and this is me, not her. She cannot feel what I'm trying to do. I start to lose the rhythm. Even dancing with the tutor, with whom I normally glide as if to the tango born, I'm unsure, staccato, stuttering.

I dance with one partner and simply have to stop.

The male instructor comes up and I say I can't feel it so I'm stepping out. He tries to tell me how to feel the beat. This never goes down well. I sit out. I slip out.

I cycle home.

As I sit on the doorstep, in the full knowledge that in a fortnight, I'll be sat in my own house, surrounded by boxes, pizza on my lap and ridiculous Bordeaux in my glass, I'm wondering.

I'm wondering why it is that now, more than ever, I need a hug.

What does it all mean? I'll tell you what it means. PD is a disease that surprises me at every turn, forces me to re-assess myself on a constant basis, to re-consider what constitutes me. One day I'm coughing and spluttering because my swallow reflex has vanished and the saliva builds up until I choke. On another day I'll be convinced I'm walking like a drunk, and I'll have to concentrate to put one foot in front of the other. On yet another day I'll be mumbling and slurring as I speak. Pick another, and I can barely move my left hand. The next day I'll have trouble getting out of bed because my muscles have stiffened up. Then I'll simply wrench a tendon because they, too, are getting ever more brittle. Then I'll feel just fine, and I'll forget. What PD means is a constant re-negotiation of the terms of engagement. Every new problem means a reassessment of behaviour, diet, excuses, lifestyle.

What PD means is that the things I enjoy will gradually become impossible for me. My life will be stripped of its meaning while, just in case that wasn't enough, I start to drool, shuffle and piss myself. PD means I'm one fucking angry sonofabitch.

But I do not, like Lear, rail against the storm. I roll with the punches. If one door closes, I bash a hole through the wall. I will be defeated, this is inevitable, but I'll be buggered if I'll roll over and let this disease tickle my tummy as it fucks me up. And I'm bloody well going to enjoy giving it the runaround. It doesn't care. There's no point personifying PD as some sort of monster, no point in doing battle with it – it simply doesn't accept your terms of engagement. My answer is not to ignore it, because that, for me, would be foolish, but to sidestep it wherever and whenever possible.

And this means a lot of sidesteps.

Earlier, I lapsed into 'them and us' terminology when discussing the reputation of PD. This is perhaps inevitable in certain situations, but I am not alone in thinking that it's less than desirable. There is, as with every interest group (and that qualifies as irony if anything does) an informal network of individuals who share PD in common. Of the few I know and speak with on a regular basis (and this may seem odd, but at the time of writing I have yet to physically meet these people, a fact that I find strange and interesting simultaneously), not one of us has the same experience of PD, nor do we treat it the same way. We veer from focused and concerted attempts to tackle it, to amass information on therapies and treatments, all the way to seemingly gay abandonment, a laugh-in-your-face treatment. Beyond the basic drug therapies, and various other straightforward modes of addressing the disease, neither end of the spectrum seems to me to have any particular advantage. PD is a disease that affects one's psychology long before it ravages the body. PD is a disease that thrives on its potential.

It wasn't the symptoms that got to me after diagnosis. If anything, diagnosis meant that I finally knew what was causing this low-level loss of fine motor control. It was an answer, it gave me some certainty. Unfortunately, as I learnt more and more about the disease and what it did, the way that it could affect my physical being, the more problems I had 'dealing with it'. When the troll under the bridge is your brain, when you are both pit and pendulum, when all the future seems to hold is a gradual but all-too-real degradation of the ability to do those things that you enjoy, that in a sense define you as an individual, then it's unsurprising that some sort of depression and perhaps erratic behaviour sets in. This is a disease that waits around the corner with a big bag of unpleasantries slung across its back in a kind of reverse swag, a malevolent Santa, doling out its gifts at random. In opposition to normal gift-giving behaviour, you know what these gifts are, just not when they're going to be doled out.

They may never come. They may all come at once. What this disease does is remove choice.

What PD can sometimes seem to mean is that you will gradually lose all sense of meaning, all sense of personality; all of the things that define and categorise you will gradually be subsumed into this one, great rolling beast of a disease. All roads lead to PD. Eventually, you will appear to the outside world (them and us again) merely as a shuffling set of symptoms. How you appear to yourself is largely up to you, but the ways in which you once defined yourself to the outside world become less and less meaningful.

I am a writer. It's what I do. At certain times of the day I can only type with one finger on my right hand. At best I can use two or three, and the third finger on my left. Voice recognition software? Well, a nice idea, but writing and speaking are very different activities, and I suspect that my voice as a writer will therefore change as I (inevitably) switch media – I may not like the idea of VR software, but this is unlikely to be a choice that I am able to make. There is, inevitably, another irony at work here. The voice (in a literal sense) that I possess at present has changed, is changing, will continue to change. It is another of the delightful effects of PD. Another of the ways in which it changes who you appear to be. But the gap between external perception and whatever 'reality' is made of really hits when revisiting an old skill, or, as in the case of the subject of this blog post, an old friend who represented an old skill.

Whole lotta shakin' … **not goin'** **on** [first published 15 Dec, 2010]

Time is a strange beast. Sometimes a straight line plummeting down into the depths, dragging us down as it goes, sometimes a great circle and we sit on the circumference watching our present, our past, and our future whizz by, just out of reach. Ok, maybe it's a spiral. The fact is, that every so often we revisit our past. Past girlfriends, past places, past lives. We know that everything will be different, yet we still strangely expect it to be the same.

Yesterday I bumped into my past, my present and my future simultaneously. And it was strange. What made it particularly strange is that while said bumping was in occurrence, I noticed that the strangeness had been noted on Facebook. 'Waiting for the Jedi master', read the status report.

I suppose I ought to explain. Yesterday, I popped out of the 'office' to visit a friend and old student. Make no mistake, this gentleman is a highly accomplished guitarist. Like me, he has trod the publishing boards, producing articles, columns and CDs for various publications. Now, I don't mind admitting that I was somewhat nervous. After all, when I was teaching him, I was über-guitarist (rock), and my every note was hung upon by students such as he. I was worried that he would dazzle me into some humility — is that it? I'm unsure.

No. I wanted to be dazzled. And I wasn't disappointed. While by his own admission a little rusty, he showed a maturity in his playing which was very impressive.

I was worried that he would think I sucked. That he would re-consider his opinion of me. That would hurt.

So, I'm explaining the Parky's and showing how frigid and rigid my left hand is (and yesterday, for some reason — tension? — it

really was pitiful) and then picked up a
guitar. Yes, I could barely string two notes
together, but there were flashes of what my
fingers could once do. I explained that so
far as I can see, actions burnt into one's
muscle memory are less affected than those
which require active nerve impulses. It's
the will which is denied by this disease.
All the same, my fingers were less than
impressive.

He fired up his amp, stuck on a backing
track, and began to wail, as they say. I
won't lie, I was itching to have a go, but
really rather scared at the possible
outcome. After all, I have hardly picked up
an electric guitar in the last ten years —
I've probably spent as long playing an
electric in that time as I used to spend in
a day practising. And to add to that, I
couldn't remember the last time I played
with an amplifier. It must be four or five
years.

So. The track finishes. He hands me his
guitar as naturally as can be, and I begin.
It's faltering at first, but my fingers
begin to loosen up just a little, and every
so often a nice little phrase pops out, or a
burning little run flies from the speakers …
in parts, my playing's really not so bad at
all.

He is very kind about the noise I'm making —
overly so, but in some ways he's right.
There is some stuff still there. Some
glimpses of what I used to be capable of.

But there is a caveat.

Every time I get to the end of a phrase — no
matter whether it's been any good or not —
my fingers simply stop. Phrasing on a guitar
is so dependent on that note, because it's

the pay-off … the note which you stamp with your personality. The note which you vibrato.

I discover something about vibrato. It doesn't live in the muscle memory. It's an instruction. You actively make the note sing.

I. Have. No. Vibrato.

This is shocking. Vibrato is one of the great levellers in guitaristic circles, and it's one of the things Parkinson's has taken away. Ironic, really. A good, good friend said on hearing of my diagnosis that I ought to get a lap steel guitar, because 'you'll have the best vibrato'. The shaking palsy, however, seems to be preventing me from shaking notes. That, children, is the true definition of irony.

Now, I know that this disease, and the therapy which accompanies it, has changed me, in some ways quite fundamentally. As a guitarist, however, it has robbed me of my identity. Bastard.

For me, the discovery that one of my old skills has vanished undermined every notion of stability I once had. Physical, intellectual, psychological … you name it, if it once seemed fixed, it now threw off its moorings and took to the high seas without so much as a by-your-leave or even the benefit of anyone at the tiller. Charts? I'm writing them now. But it's also so much bigger than this.

As we navigate our way through life, we see bad things happening. Really bad things, those cataclysmic events that scar entire generations tend not to happen in England. And so, when there's a tsunami or an epidemic, we feel sympathy, the government sends condolences, and sometimes, if we're feeling a little flush, we send a little cash (or maybe some old clothes), and we consider our duty discharged. So far as I can see, we don't really care. What really goes through our heads is 'rather you than me', and we give to cover up the fact that in the grand scheme of things we do nothing. Charity is selfish. This, however, doesn't make it bad ... to me, it's the pretence that is, the philanthropic pose. Sometimes we need to accept that we're selfish, and even work on the principle that being selfish, or, at least, looking to yourself first, can actually be the most productive and useful thing all around.

When Lisbon was destroyed by a massive earthquake in the eighteenth century, leading to almost unimaginable casualties within hours, it triggered an inordinate amount of soul-searching and discussion. What it all came down to was whether a truly loving god could allow this terrible disaster to happen. When the discussion reached this point, the horror was not at what had happened to the people of Lisbon, but what the implications were for the world. After all, it appeared that one of the more troublesome interpretations of the earthquake was that God was, at best, sleeping on duty. This was unthinkable, so it wasn't long before it became almost acceptable to doubt the very existence of god, and the next question which raised its ugly head was, if there is no god, 'what does it all mean?'

We give to charity to salve our soul and to avoid having to address the question. Like many if not all of us, there have been times when I've truly failed to see the point of it all. Not being one of the faithful, one of those who can attach themselves and their meaning to some nebulous 'creator' (devastating earthquakes notwithstanding), I find myself forced to manufacture my life's meaning all by myself. It does make things more awkward, but it's just the way it is. The upside is the lack of self-delusion; the downside the lack of self-delusion. When things get tough, you've really got no-one but yourself to rely on. No-one else to lean on.

So, diagnosis. This is a process of external examination. This has already happened, and while it involves an awful lot of input on the part of the patient, especially with a clinical diagnosis such as is demanded by a condition like PD, it is fundamentally controlled from the outside. Diagnosis is an imposition. It is given to you. Impositions such as this are the kind that make you stop and ask yourself what exactly is going on.

It took me a fair while to realise that the really big question had not actually been answered. In fact, it hadn't really been asked. PD is a progressive condition, and as it progresses it takes you with it. The questions it asks are many and continuous.

PD means continually having to adjust to and, in certain situations, pre-empt the worst effects. It's seeing that as your body and mind gradually change, you have to choose whether to change with it, to ignore it, or to give in to it.

First, I ignored it. I knew what it was, and what it did, after all. PD has a reputation, but how did my experience square with it? During the active part of PD, that is, when you're actively being diagnosed or actively telling people, there's little time to think. When the hullaballoo dies down a little, you start to consider those questions people ask, or want to ask, such as 'what does it mean for you?' Sometimes they pretty much hit the nail on the head, sometimes they're way off base. Whichever extreme they hit, whichever meaning they ascribe to your PD, it makes you think … and it makes you take a position. Furthermore, the disease slowly permeates your world, and after diagnosis the possible or likely paths of the disease have a serious impact on how you make medium to long-term plans.

But the disease really does do strange things. What's perhaps strangest is the way in which you discover this. I know my gait is getting worse. I can feel it as I walk. It's awkward, and my left leg drags sometimes, and sometimes it just falls flap on to the ground, and other times the toes get caught in the pavement. Walking on uneven surfaces, or where the slope is left to right, is really uncomfortable.

I had a minor revelation the other day. I walk strangely because my left foot doesn't actually know where the ground is. This may sound odd (well, that's because it is odd) but it's perfectly logical. You simply don't know until you lose the foot radar that this is what's happening. And it wasn't my gait that told me that I had a problem with my ability to sense the position of this ball of rock atop which we sit. No. It was an experiment. An experiment with a therapy recommended by a fellow PWP: banging on a set of drums. Like most of us, I imagine, I'm resistant when it comes to advice if it comes from someone whose experience of PD is limited to a news item or two, which then apparently gives them the right to join the medical profession, and patronise the PWP. This happens all the time ... one was when the National Ballet were 'doing ballet' with a roomful of PWP, and the next thing you hear is that ballet is the new wonder-therapy. Frankly, this gets stale very, very quickly.

I tend to react quite instinctively to such news, placing it firmly into the box marked 'celebrity toss'. I'm all for publicising and raising funds and trying to act on the subject of a cure, and I have no problem with people using their name when they have some connection with PD. When someone says that we shouldn't treat PWP as freaks it's bad enough (we are actually real people, apparently), but when that person starts speaking about something they are paid to promote as a therapy then I cannot help but smell the whiff of cynical cashing-in. Invariably, these sorts of studies don't register on the radars of non-sufferers (Or how to say it? Non-afflicted? Non-diseased?).

As with everything, you become just that little bit more attuned when something affects you directly, and spot the platitudes and straightforward errors propagated by lazy journalism. What's more, you begin to see how the manner in which things are reported has a very serious impact on people's attitude towards others. It's obvious, yes, but that doesn't stop us from ignoring it until it happens to us. The following blog post was an exasperated reaction to one such news 'feature' on TV.

A curate's omelette [first published 13 June, 2012]

I'm always part open, part suspicious when people start saying to me, 'so, %&$$£** is the new cure for Parkinson's'. Open because I want, unsurprisingly, for there to be something new to report … suspicious, because I fear another Helen Mirren Wii-fit patronisefest. Last night's Inside Out London pushed both buttons for me, and has led to endless tutu jokes doing the rounds. I have no problem with tutus, by the way. I immediately saw one problem … that is, there was no-one young in this group. For PD, young means under fifty … those early-onsetters like myself who were diagnosed at or before the age of forty.

The programme is presented by some bloke who says things like 'What's great about this is that I can see that they're genuinely having a good time, dancing, moving and expressing themselves, not thinking at all about Parkinson's.' Well, let me point out that 'they' is patronising (he means 'those ill, old people, not young hotties like me'), I'm not convinced simply following the moves of one part of the Nutcracker is 'expressing themselves' so much as expressing the choreographer and Tchaikovsky, and how in god's name do you know they're 'not thinking at all about Parkinson's'. Sorry. Dick. There. I've said it. Furthermore, his commentary reminds me of nothing less than a natural history programme.

The casually good-looking Dr Sarah Houston (you see, I can do it too) is much better when she talks of PWP doing movements that are different, and she's right, but I can't help but feel a teensy bit of 'pull yourselves together' about her when she says 'actually what you're doing is feeling different'. Now, this all seems to be a bit stating-the-bleedin-obvious. Of course movement will help, and of course that's great. But it all seems so obvious to me.

Psychologically, we do not like to do stuff we find hard or are bad at. Directed movement for the PWP is hard, and you're not very good at it. The result is, naturally, that we move less, and the less we move, the less able we are to move. It's a self-fulfilling, self-affecting prophecy. Now then. Here's the science bit. Anything that gets a PWP moving is going to have a positive effect on the patient. Because it will turn back the secondary effect of PD, which is to limit movement. So of course getting Jane and John (you see what I did there?) to do anything is going to help everything work better.

But then the feature gets lazy again. The presenter opines thus about Jane, mostly wheelchair-bound: 'In spite of her condition, dancing has always been a part of her life.' Er, hang on a second, she was diagnosed in 2005. She is older than 6, therefore, forgive me, but this sort of lazy writing just patronises. It's also illogical and pointless. I do wonder why Jane thought she'd never be able to express herself in dance again though she had been a keen dancer throughout her life. Is this because as she became clumsier, stiffer, no-one would dance with her? Or was it because she couldn't face dancing badly, when she had, I imagine, once been accomplished? If the former, for shame. If the latter, for shame on no-one organising therapeutic dance sessions. Oh, hang on … they have?

I don't want all this to end up as yet another Chinese-whisper stylee 'cure' for PD. But I do think that it's a great thing. But I find it hard to pick one dance over another. Don't fret about the style — anything formalised yet fluid and non-rigid will suffice, I shouldn't wonder. Or perhaps style should fit age and advancement … but then again, tango is fabulous, I have found, and in many ways it mirrors the sorts of movements that martial arts have, which can also be very beneficial to the PWP. Sarah talks about measurable improvements, and that's great. It's also no surprise to me. Anything which makes a PWP do stuff will help. Because when we do stuff our body understands, we're fine. It's when our brain has to get in the way and send instructions to our various body parts that we're in trouble.

This is where, as ever, everything gets wishy-washy … there's no real talk of how and why it will help, and especially odd is the lack of conclusion with regards preventative care — I'm sure martial arts or dance classes for the newly diagnosed, when delivered on the NHS as a matter of course, would save hundreds of thousands of pounds in the long run … and make for much happier patients.

There were some useful insights, mind, the talk of rhythm helping walking is interesting, as is Sarah's use of the word 'stutter' — this is actually quite an accurate portrayal of how PD feels sometimes (to me, anyway). My instinct suggests that the point behind 'feeling the rhythm' is that this takes the mind away from the problem at hand, while making the body work as a whole.

The thing with dance and sport and martial arts is that they strengthen the body and make it work as a machine rather than a bundle of individual parts which don't really talk to one another. This is what helps us function better, when our limbs work in concert, not against one another.

And this is what amazes me. The fact that no-one seems to have thought to ask a PWP their opinions. Because, to be frank, we're way ahead of you on this one. Bloody talk to us. We're not them, we're people. With names. And it isn't just Parkinson's.

When it comes to this disease, I, along with many of my contemporaries, find it far more helpful to listen to an actual sufferer than an expert or the more usual 'I saw a programme on it and this is what you should do' sort of advice. This is because, as I've said, PD is a very personal condition. It's not a one-size-fits-all problem, not in terms of medication, nor in terms of therapy. Most therapies offer temporary symptomatic relief, that is, they make you feel better for a bit. There's nothing wrong with temporary unless you think it's permanent. So with PD I don't struggle where struggle is pointless, but that's a very different thing from ignoring the disease in the forlorn hope that it will go away. I listen with arms folded to most people on the subject of PD, but pay attention when fellow PWPs say that something has helped. One of the daftest but most fabulous PWP of my acquaintance recently took up drumming. She swears by it. So much so that she has begun a campaign to get drummers to lend us their kits (oops, you see, this 'them and us' business is catching, apparently). Her basic premise is that hitting things in a rhythmic manner helps. Helps her focus. Helps her forget.

I can think of many reasons why drumming could be useful therapy for PWP, but perhaps the most interesting is the psychological effect of hitting something with a stick and its going BOOM! This is because PWP in general don't make enough noise – they are often softly spoken because of the disease itself, and tend not to make wild demonstrative gestures either – and making noise really helps to connect you with the world in a visceral sense: hitting drums makes you feel quite alive. It's very cause and effect. I instinctively understood this, but thought it would be interesting to see what it *felt* like. Whether I got what she got.

So, I cracked open my address book (ok, I opened Facebook), and messaged one Mike Sturgis, erstwhile head of drums at the Academy of Contemporary Music in Guildford and regular Rhythm magazine contributor. Now, Mike and I used to teach at the Musician's Institute/London Music School in Wapping back in the 90s, and we'd often get to play together, demonstrating tunes at music shows, that sort of thing. I am not flattering him when I say that he is the man – quite simply my favourite drummer to play with (and I've been lucky enough to play with Thomas Lang, considered by many to be the best there is). There's a good reason for this, and it's not that he's a lovely chap (which he is), but that his groove is so big and fat and utterly there that it acts like a small planet, pulling your own notes into its centre through some sort of rhythmic gravity. You not only can't go wrong, but you can go way outside the norm rhythmically and not slip up on his beat. He really does rock.

So, I contacted him with mixed feelings. He didn't know about my diagnosis, so there was a little awkwardness when we spoke on the phone The journey to his teaching studio was also a little fraught. It was as if I was journeying to my past. Things I perhaps didn't want to be reminded of were about to leap up and bite me.

He was drumming when I entered the room.

Mike and I greeted each other and chatted a bit. Rather nervously.

Frankly, I felt odd, and didn't want to make a complete tit of myself. But I gritted my teeth and sat behind a kit for the first time in years and years ... and years. Picked up a stick and hit the bloody thing.

Now. Let's get a few things straight. Playing the drums is hard. I mean, it's easy in a certain sense. The sense in which you take a stick and hit big things and they make a noise. In that sense it's a doddle. I'm sitting on the drum stool with a drummer I have intense respect for watching my every move. And he knows what sort of knowledge I bring to this particular table. The sort of knowledge that acts as a great inhibitor. But it's time to get over myself. Time to play some drums and see what all the fuss is about.

I already know that I'll approach drumming-as-therapy differently to my friend, simply because PD has hit us differently. Partly this is because she has had a year or two more of it, and partly because we're just different people.

So. I start with technique. It's what I understand. The grip. How to hold the sticks. The right hand is quite orthodox but the left hand is (unsurprisingly) recalcitrant. I struggle with orthodox grip, so I try 'match grip', the funny sideways grip you see in marching bands. This sort of works, but I soon swap back, though I tend to use the arm rather than wrist in the left wing, but eventually fix this by twisting my hand more. It is, naturally, quite difficult and takes some concentration. It is at this point that I notice the first oddness, the first indication that things aren't going to run quite as smoothly as I'd like.

My left-hand stick has two faults. The first is the fact that it scoops at the drum head rather than going straight down and straight up – this means it glances the skin rather than hitting it square, with the obvious lack of sonic pleasingness. The second is perhaps more of a problem, and more difficult to diagnose. My stick doesn't know where the drum head is.

This may sound like a rather surreal problem, but it's of vital importance for groove that the player knows exactly where the dead centre of the note is. Perhaps a sporting analogy will help. When kicking a football, the foot must kick through the line of the dead centre of the ball if it is to go straight. Any slight deviation from this plain means that the ball will begin to spin just a little, altering its trajectory. As with balls, so with notes. The player who knows where the note's centre is can control the note at will. The drummer is the player who provides the unifying 'this is where the big, fat, juicy centre of the groove resides' for the band, and the fatter the centre, the bigger the groove.

The thing with grooves, and tight-as bands, is that everyone knows where this note-centre is. As a guitarist or bass-player, you have to predict where the note-centre is, so you can lock in with the drummer. Groove is a predictive art, and when everyone concludes that it's in the same place, greatness results. The great drummer leaves you in no doubt as to where the note-centre is going to explode, so everyone hits it with ease (that's what Mike does, by the way).

My left hand doesn't know where the drum head is … which is going to make co-ordination practically impossible …

You see, sometimes I know too much. I don't blindly and blithely blunder ahead, full of confidence and blarney. Not I. I see what's around the corner and wonder whether I ought not turn left instead of right.

But we press on. I play straight four, with eights on the hi-hat, adding stuff until I'm playing eights on the ride, quarters on the hi-hat via the pedal, kick/snare on the 1 and 3/2 and 4 respectively. Add some fills, stick in a tom roll or two … and we're away.

The big question is: does it make a difference? Well, how can I tell? I did no dexterity tests beforehand to make a later comparison with, though I noticed afterwards that I could flick change out of my left palm with my thumb, which is normally impossible (though I wouldn't have been able to feed a parking meter). But I'll happily state that my being felt more at ease with itself afterwards. This makes me wonder whether a) I shouldn't start keeping a PD journal with relatively objective tests within, and b) whether music, and especially rhythm, helps. Certainly I know that the tango is useful. I shy away from the PDJ because, as I said to Mike, I don't want a graph of my life as it ebbs away. I don't want to make myself a mere point of study. I don't want to mechanise myself, to turn myself into a statistic voluntarily. This would not do at all. Sometimes, it's enough that the world wants to make me into a patient, and I don't see why I ought to help it.

What was all this leading to? Well, it was the realisation that my left hand couldn't work out where the drum head was that allowed me to understand that my gait was becoming increasingly challenging because my feet didn't know where the floor was.

Currently, it seems, PD is working to disassociate my self from myself. My body seems to be detaching itself not so much from my mind, but from my instincts ... my emotions, even. I watch concerts and feel nothing. And yet, on the way to my drum lesson, I was singing along to a Tom Baxter tune (Skybound, would you warrant it?), and I began to cry. Tears. In floods. Here's a musing on this very subject:

Emotional anaesthesia [first published 28 March, 2012]

Last night I went to a concert at the Brighton Dome. It was the Waterboys, ostensibly flogging the new album, An Appointment with Mr Yeats. Now, the album is pretty good, and Mike Scott's free interpretation of Yeats' poetry creates something a little more than the sum of all its parts. His cherry-picking of lines from various poems may offend the purist, but in many ways is close to the spirit of Yeats' own work, as he played wild and loose with Ireland's mythic past.

Let's face it, if you can't play wild and loose with myth, something's very wrong.

Now I'm a dreadful gig-goer, as I'm wildly critical, knowing as I do a little about the process. This is compounded by an increasing susceptibility to sleep when rhythmic stuff is happening. Put me on a train and I'm asleep in minutes, my head dipping, probably accompanied by muttering and foaming at the mouth. I had terrible trouble at a gig I was reviewing once, but somehow I heard everything even while asleep. Lucky escape. The trend for 'older' bands to show off their ability to stand up while their audience sit down and mutter if any of their neighbours dare to show any sense of interest in proceedings doesn't help matters.

So, last night was difficult from the get-go … that and there were issues of a sonic variety. Mike Scott's mic was uber-sibilant and distorting a little, and the sound in general was poor — though part of this is attributable to our position on the stage-right of the horseshoe that is the circle. The band, I thought, were poor. The drummer and the bass player apparently felt the beat in different places, one ahead of it, the other behind. Not a good thing. Mike Scott himself paced the stage in a most equine fashion, pawing at the ground with his hooves in what was probably affected fashion once but has now I suspect become simply the way he plays.

The band simply played their parts without any real connection between themselves, and nothing with the audience whatsoever. Well, they utterly failed to connect with me, that's for sure.

But I'm beginning to wonder whether something else is going on here. Last night I felt emotionally disconnected; numb. I couldn't feel anything. Though I could feel my skin. This is a particularly strange phenomenon. I have yet to understand it.

While I was feeling nothing but the flexible covering which envelops me, my eyes closed and I drifted off. It's as if the lack of connection had switched me off — either that or I switched off and thus had no connection available. Which came first …

So, in a chicken and egg situation, one takes the sensible route — the exit. Why sit nodding off when it inhibits the enjoyment of your companions? I left during the interval.

I am beginning to wonder whether this bloody disease is partly culpable. I do seem to be having connectivity issues. Just as my brain has trouble connecting with my left hand, and often my left leg, so my emotional centres seem as if they've been bypassed. There may well be a whole host of women now shaking their heads and going 'no shit', but it's not that simple.

Nothing's ever that simple.

As I left the venue, I shuffled rather than walked … and recently I've noticed my gait becoming more compromised. Furthermore, I've been looking at chapter four, ostensibly on the attempt to find meaning in the disease, and I've realised that I don't have a clue. What it all means. More than that, however, I don't even know how to articulate my inability to ascribe it meaning.

I currently feel considerably less than the sum of my parts.

Perhaps this is what PD means to me – it means that I must do rather than merely experience. I find reading nigh-on impossible these days. But I write a lot.

It makes some sort of perverse sense.

Full of wise saws –
on making a plan of action

What next? After it all starts to settle, the dust of diagnosis and the realisation that you've turned some sort of corner, the sort with an invisible turnstile such that once you've been through there is no coming back, the thorny question of the future starts to set in. While prognosis for PD is generally better for those diagnosed young, it's only a relative thing. The standard fifteen-year life expectancy from diagnosis is rather conservative for the early-onset patient. In terms of physical effects, it's also not that great, as prognoses go … a gradual though marked decline in the faculties, a loss of control of the body. The removal of choice. The first thing you're offered, naturally, is chemical intervention.

The drugs [don't] work?

The song is palpably untrue. They do. I have felt it. It is rather difficult to judge their efficacy because of the way one of the most common family of drugs used to treat the symptoms of PD (and symptomatic control is all that can be achieved), dopamine agonists, must be delivered. They are designed to stimulate the production of dopamine in the cells still alive. The dosage is personal. The drug must be titrated, that is, introduced in small dosages which are increased gradually until the required level is reached – a level dictated by results. Coming off drugs such as the one I currently take is no simple matter. You must wean your brain off it slowly, so any change of function is also gradual. The large leaflet that accompanies these tablets makes this plain:

If you suffer from Parkinson's disease you should not stop treatment with _____ abruptly. A sudden stop could cause you to develop a medical condition called neuroleptic malignant syndrome which may represent a major health risk. The symptoms include:

akinesia (loss of muscle movement),
rigid muscles,
fever,
unstable blood pressure,
tachycardia (increased heart rate),
confusion,
depressed level of consciousness (e.g. coma).

It's the beautiful understatement that I love: 'e.g. coma'. That's quite depressed in terms of consciousness, I reckon. One up from that very depressed level they call death …

But some drugs, such as levodopa, can be taken in one hit. One of the secondary tests for PD is, or was, seeing if levodopa actually works. Levodopa is a metabolic precursor of dopamine, synthesised from Tyrosine, an amino acid. It's the gold standard treatment for PD, but has several small issues of its own that mean it's generally saved for when things 'get bad'. In short, levodopa as a therapy has a limited period of efficacy. It works for around five years, and then it's done. This leads the PWP down a rather thorny path, as at some point, the decision will have to be made. It's a simple enough question, but like all simple questions, it's an incredibly tough one to answer. The difficulty is in working out when to start taking it to provide maximum benefit. Is this later on, when the symptoms are particularly bad, and the drug will roll them back to a far less unpleasant level, though an unknown one, naturally? Or is it to be taken early, in order to keep the PWP as close to 'normal' for as long as possible, accepting that when the drug loses its efficacy, the decline may be quite marked.

The almost wittily named 'levodopa challenge' is simple. You do stuff. You take (a lot of) levodopa. You do it again. If the difference is marked, that's another reason to think that your diagnosis of PD was correct.

I was sent off to complete this 'challenge' a year or so after my initial diagnosis. I was told that I would complete 'a battery' of physical tests, take the levodopa, (rinse) and repeat. I was not to take my morning dose of Mirapexin, allowing the dopamine agonist to run out overnight, the better to contrast the before and after of the levodopa. All interesting so far. I was warned that levodopa often caused nausea and sometimes vomiting when given suddenly in high doses (as it was to be), so I was prescribed an anti-emetic.

To be honest, I was pretty scared. I'm not entirely sure why. Then I was confused when I read that the anti-emetic was a dopamine agonist ... surely some mistake? But a phone call to my then girlfriend confirmed that it would not affect the test. In typical fashion, my stressed self had read incorrectly, as the anti-emetic, Domperidone, is a dopamine *ant*agonist. It's no surprise I misread.

I sat in the waiting room/arse end of the neurology ward, waiting. I had blood taken by a very cute nurse, which made me feel much better, as a good flirt always does. Then a plain-clothes medic strolled in, asking if I was Dr Langman. I nodded and she asked me to follow her. Ah, I thought, the neurological testing suite. Perfect. I had an intellectual interest in the tests they would put me through. After all, I had already designed some of my own, in idle moments.

She led me into the busy ward corridor. 'See that mark?' she pointed to a red mark on the wall. I nodded. 'Stay here [why bother with the mark?] and when I say go, walk naturally towards me.' I did so. She walked back to the first red mark (after making me wait at a second), and I walked again. 'It's quite mild, then,' she said. It was practically an accusation. Now that's a strange sensation, feeling as if you're being robbed of your patient status ... the status you rail against so often. We went back to the waiting room. I was confused. She took a piece of A4 out of her handbag and flattened it, then drew two round dots about 6 inches apart. She told me to point to each in turn with my index finger until she said stop. I did this with both hands.

Then she handed me a pill. 'Take this'. I stared at her. 'Is that it?' She nodded. I swallowed. She vanished. I waited.

Three quarters of an hour later, I repeated the tests. I walked one second quicker. I forget the number of times I hit the spots in a minute, but with the drug both hands were pretty evenly matched, unlike before, when the left hand had lagged behind.

'This is all a bit pointless, you know, because I know what you're doing.'

'You're trying to do it quicker?' She looked horrified.

'No,' I replied, 'but now I know what you're looking for, the test ceases to be of much use.' It seemed obvious that once I realised the test was reliant on my continuing to behave naturally, I was in trouble. It's similar to those times when a dentist or suchlike says 'just relax'. You know something's about to happen. Something you don't like. Relaxing is just about the last thing you're likely to do.

I left the clinic utterly fucking furious. So much so that I strode to the parking machine (still racks me off having to pay to park to get prodded ... leaving after being diagnosed it seemed like pouring salt into the wound) and grabbed the money out of my left-hand pocket while dialling with my right hand. I fed the machine, flicking coins from the palm of my hand with my thumb into the slot. As the machine whirred, it hit me: I can't do this. Usually, I have enough trouble getting anything out of my left-hand pocket. It causes untold embarrassment as I reach around with my right to help manoeuvre keys or coins into my left hand and try to grasp. It looks, I suspect, like I'm playing with my cock. I'm sure if I were twenty years older and drooling just a little, I would be accused of all manner of things as, hand shaking, I delve deep into my trousers and fiddle impotently. Just to make things worse, my hand often freezes in my pocket, and I simply can't get it out. I struggle for a while before either lifting up my entire left arm at the shoulder, or reach around with my right hand and yank it out.

'Fuck me, this shit *works*!' I said as the phone at the other end was picked up. 'The tests were shit. Why the fuck they didn't ask me what I thought about this levodopa shit is beyond me.'

And so it seems the patient/doctor dichotomy widens.

This is what PD means. It means no-one asks. Apart from when they can only ask. Making plans for this is hard. How can you plan for something that won't happen? Pretty much the only option is to become rather more proactive than you might like, and then ... well, what happens is simple. You proactively talk about your disease, you take command of the few parts of PD that are susceptible to being commanded. And these parts are yourself. And all the while you repeat the mantra 'I am not my condition'.

The other confirmatory test, that is, one which is less a diagnostic tool than a way of reinforcing the PD decision, is the DAT scan. This involves radioactive gunk and a big electromagnet which circles the head for thirty minutes. Stay away from children and animals for a week, and your piss might, well, glow (metaphorically speaking). But that's right. Half a bleedin' hour. No headcase here, just a rather ineffectual strap, and a warning not to move or they'll have to rescan. I lost all sense of time, kept falling asleep, waking in a panic thinking I'd done the jerking limb on dropping off thing. No isolation, no real clue what was going on. When I was told to wait until they checked I hadn't moved, I didn't know whether I had been flat out for three, thirteen or thirty minutes. But it was the letter which astounded me. It began thus:

We are delighted ...

Delighted? To tell me that yes, it is my brain cracking up? That I do have impaired dopamine uptake, blah, blah, blah? This modern obsession with being positive and personal sometimes gets out of hand. Though there is some logic at work here, even if it is rather skewed ...

PD is a personal disease. Its progression, its symptoms, its attitude, all of these are different (within certain parameters, naturally) for each individual, and so it's difficult, if not impossible, to make plans. Furthermore, when you do take steps to prevent something uncertain, something that you cannot know will happen, you can only know the effectiveness of your actions if they fail (if you do not wish your kitten to eat the robin in your back garden, you may put a bell on its collar. If it then does not eat the robin, it may simply be that it has no hunger for such a treat. If, however, the kitten trots back into the house with a red-breasted corpse in its mouth, then you can be sure that the bell has failed in its mission). Considering these issues, the question surely is less 'how do you make plans?' than it is 'why bother making plans at all?'

More questions than answers, this disease. That's certainly something that I'm getting used to. I'm also getting progressively more used to surprises. More than anything, I'm understanding that it's becoming increasingly difficult to separate the effects of the disease from those of its drug therapies. As there's no cure, we rely on symptomatic relief, and those things that we rely on to ameliorate the symptoms contribute to the sum total of things that trouble us. Among the many optional extras is the hallucination. It's something that is perhaps under-reported, for reasons that will become increasingly plain. Earlier this year, I was driving from Scotland to Brighton, through the driving rain (which was driving in the opposite direction and on the wrong side of the road), when something very strange happened. Something very strange indeed. Here's what I wrote on my blog.

There be spiders [first published 24 Feb, 2012]

'It's very interesting,' I noted during an early morning chat with a fellow PD-wrangler, as she recounted her first, and rather scary, hallucination. Interesting because her brain had chosen to inject life into a hat and scarf hanging on the back of a door, so much so that she had been forced to touch it, to confirm with one sense what her intellect knew and yet her sight denied. Interesting because we suffer from a brain-based movement disorder which makes our bodies move uncontrollably, or makes it difficult to control our bodies. Why the projection of movement on to inanimate objects? Why translate this movement as a sign of life rather than of the wind?

The physical parts of PD are in themselves rather unsettling, sometimes scary, eventually debilitating, but it is perhaps the stuff that goes on inside the head which is most interesting, if possibly in a Chinese sense. Eventually, everyone can see you have PD, but it's the stuff contained in our own little personal prison, our own lifelong solitary confinement, which is really crippling.

I have been hallucinating for some time. Nothing major. No great rends in the fabric of reality, no rips in the space-time continuum, just small, mild, unsettling things. The most common is the 'horror movie scuttling things' hallucination. When the protagonists are still unaware of their fate, they often pick up flashes of darkness, mainly flashing (if darkness may be allowed to flash) across open doorways. I do the same to myself, creating things in my peripheral vision, things which are palpably there, but not there. Schrödinger's things. Looking collapses the hallucination. These used to worry me, now they're almost comforting — reminders of what I am that stay internal, so that no-one else can see.

I, too, have a thing about making things alive. I tend not to create movement, but to mistranslate movement as a sign of life. I once watched a spider scuttle backwards and forward in a short elliptical pattern on the bathroom floor for about a minute, trying to work out its motivation. It was almost as if it was playing out the stress patterns you see in caged animals where they grind a path

into the earth as they walk, repeat; walk,
repeat. Eventually I realised that this
spider was merely the shadow of the thing on
the end of the bathroom light pull cord.

Unless you're particularly scared of
spiders, this isn't the most perturbing of
hallucinations possible, but it's the
principle. Why is it that the brain decides
to mislead me this way? Why, and this is
perhaps more pertinent, do I insist on
granting my brain its own will? What
possesses me to think that the grey matter
is purposely fucking with my mind?
This is perhaps the greatest hallucination
of them all: the personification of the
brain. Disease is not aware. It does not
have feelings. It does not make decisions.
PD is not a dragon you can fight. There's no
challenging something that doesn't recognise
your rules. My brain is neither for nor
against me. It merely is. It's just that
some of it has merrily wandered off into its
own territory.

There be spiders there.

What happened in the car was far worse than merely inventing
a spider to explain a moving shadow that otherwise doesn't
compute. The windscreen wiper turned into a human arm. It
traversed its upwards trajectory as a perfectly normal
windscreen wiper, but on the way down it was an arm. In a
sleeve. My windscreen wiper turned into a human arm. The
sleeve was that of an anorak. Well, you're not going to go out
in the lashing rain wearing a T-shirt, now are you? I freaked
for a split second. As you can imagine. It was a bit like having
an eye-test when they check the pressure of the eyeball with a
puff of compressed air – you know it's coming but your

reflexes still kick in. Knowledge in this case is of no real use. So with the arm. Knowing that I occasionally hallucinate, and that when I do it takes the form of breathing life into inanimate objects, did not make one iota of difference to my reaction. Even if I'd known the hallucinations could be so vivid, it would still have been one of shock.

How can one plan in the face of a disease for which the therapy can have such diverse effects, even within the same category? Scuttling shapes in the peripheral vision to windscreen wipers turning into arms. Both are hallucinations, but they hardly come under the same category. This you cannot prepare for. What you can do is accelerate the process of assimilation. To do this, you need to know what to expect.

It isn't what you think. Now, this is where things get, well … juicy. There's no easy way to say this stuff. The drugs work on more than just the PD. There's a set of traits associated with dopamine agonists that are perhaps more common than the side-effect sheets lead you to believe. Put simply, they can accentuate obsessive behaviour, while simultaneously sending your attention span into terminal decline.

It's a delicious irony, in fact, that the obsessive behaviour – cataloguing, organising and so on – is balanced so beautifully with an inability to stick with the cataloguing, organising, and so on. My laptop is full of to-do lists, tables and plans. I do the list, and then before I've finished I'm doing another. I've gone from being highly organised, anally retentive some might say, to filing things in a pile. I lose things, I forget things, and yet I obsess about my keys. I check whether I have my keys with me relentlessly. I talk to myself about them. My keys are in my top left-hand pocket. Right. Where are my keys? Top left-hand pocket. Am I sure? Well, I'd better check. Oh. They're not there. Let's check every pocket. Oh dear. Let's check again.

Top left-hand pocket. Excellent, they there are. Now, where did I put them again? This behaviour obviously isn't limited to those on agonists, but, dammit, I never used to behave like this.

I usually get my keys out a hundred or so yards from my house. Then I put them back. All the while I'm talking quietly about what I need to do next. Like a mantra. Even I think I'm strange, sometimes. Currently the most common way I address myself is with the words 'what I need is ...'

And yet, this obsessive behaviour is not merely balanced by an inability to finish things, it also comes with a compulsive element. This compulsive behaviour, for me, takes two distinct forms. The first is wrapped up with the obsessive streak, and is in many ways akin to an addiction, but I'll save that until after we look at the gung-ho compulsion.

At its most benign, the gung-ho compulsion can actually be seen as a good thing. It is, I suspect, a combination of the drugs whispering 'do it, do it' in my ear, and the simple acceptance that this bastard disease is slowly but surely taking away my choices. Every week, every month, every year that goes by sees some loss – and not only is this loss greater than the simple act of ageing, but it starts from a point of lesser ability. This year, 2012, has so far been quite depressing for me, as my simple physicality has taken a hit in the shape of a shoulder operation, an operation undertaken to fix a trauma whose roots can be traced directly back to PD. I ripped it in training, while I was practicing a jujitsu-based martial art. I ripped it because I did something stupid, something stubborn, the effects of which were accentuated by one of the more hidden symptoms of PD. The disease causes your tendons to become brittle and your muscles to stiffen. This in turn contributes to the slowness of movement you see in PWP, and makes injury more likely, as stiff muscles and brittle tendons fail to deal with certain physical acts as they should. The shock absorbers rust up. The impact goes directly to the bit that is usually protected.

That's the physical bit.

Mix gung-ho compulsion with the realisation of just how short my useful life may be and the injury makes more sense.

Yes, I know this is miserable. Yes, I know this is hard to read. But it's hard to live, too, and it's hard to work out how to live. It's hard to watch. It's hard to see other people watching it, watching you experience it.

I mentioned this at the beginning. I'm not expecting you to enjoy this book. I'm merely hoping that it may be helpful. I'm guessing that by now you've sort of guessed the intention behind the structure, the reality of the narrative flow. The seven ages are also my moods. It starts with utter naiveté, runs through inability to comprehend into simple disbelief, before defiance turns into anger.

Back to the gung-ho compulsion

It seems to work like this. At some point (and it's usually quite quickly, if my highly partial straw poll is anything to go by), the PWP realises that those things he or she enjoys now come with a 'best before' date. These are usually things that the PWP takes as part of their identity. I am a cricketer, for example. I am painfully aware that my usefulness as a cricketer is limited at best, as the PD causes a couple of problems that really get in the way. Slowness of movement. Difficulty moving the feet. Weakening grip. These three things have meant that my cricket has declined in relative terms over the past three years, and I've only kept it there or thereabouts through hard work.

I've known the PD has been affecting my play for the past two years, and so I made a conscious decision: to play as much as I can, while I can.

This often translates as playing through injury, choosing game over work, saying yes before any specific consequences are considered. Taking it too seriously.

I see things getting worse. It hits me every so often – increasingly often, to be fair. Generally, in some unexpected place, at an unexpected time, an unexpected thing occurs. It can be something as simple as my holding out my hand or pointing a finger. I begin to tremor. Increasingly, someone notices. When I stand at the non-striker's end after a quick single, my right hand often loses itself in a blur of shudder and judder. Pouring milk into coffee. Holding a casserole dish whose lid isn't quite right. Oftentimes, it simply manifests in a lethargy that makes others tut in exasperation. Here are my thoughts regarding one such incident, again from my blog.

Milestones and millstones [first published May 2012]

Every so often you see them. Fingerposts. They point the way not merely with a sign but with a finger, like the manicules you find in old books, red hands in the margin pointing to some salient piece of information. They're old, and ragged, and not necessarily particularly accurate as indicators of just how far one has to travel to reach one's destinations. They are similar in many ways to the semi-pyramidal stones one sees which assert one's position, yet these are accurate to within seconds, geographically speaking. Both indicators of position, relative or absolute, pale somewhat in the face of the humble smartphone, which happily tells you where you're at wherever you're at — there is no need to wait.

Today I found myself both fingerposted and milestoned, placenamed and satnavved. Irritatingly, it took place at Sainsbury's. When checking out, the personage always (but always) asks whether you need any help packing. For years this has irritated me, as even though I know that it's a thing they must do, it still makes me think they think I'm incapable. For years I've made a joke about it, complained at their professionalism, how they outrun me so easily. Naturally, they pack a bag.

I do this because they're so bloody quick. In the old days, the days when going to the supermarket meant having twelve pounds and seventeen pence and counting as you filled your basket, the checkouters had to tap everything in by hand. You could keep up easily. Now it's all super-efficient, but the shopper remains the same.

Today, she didn't ask. The couple behind me (the male half of which berated his partner when she smiled at me as we acknowledged the bloody torturous screaming of several children in the vicinity — there were about ten. All screaming. Yowzer) waited as I packed. Or tried to.

It starts with the bags. My fingers don't want to open them. The items stack up.

It continues with the holding open of the bag while placing items in. My left hand starts to shake. The aperture of the bag changes, my right hand joins in. The bottle of wine/juice/whatever hovers shakily and catches the edges of the bag.

The items stack up.

They begin to form a very disorderly queue, tumbling like rockfall, the terminal moraine of a glacier of groceries. My hands shake ever more as I see them stack up. I feel the opprobrium of the couple behind me. I slowly fill my three bags full. I have no wool, just woolly limbs, ever descending into uselessness.

I am yanked back to the day of initial diagnosis, when I had gone straight from neurology to nurturing students, lecturing on the Fairie Queene. I had wanted to scream at the assembled throng, in between talk of the Redcrosse Knight and Duessa's fowl dugs and loins askirt with foxes, or whatever: 'I've got fucking Parkinson's. FUCK!'

I didn't. Either time.

Every so often, something happens that reminds me not only that I'm ill, but that I'm getting iller. Milestones become millstones.

One day, I'll simply drown.

I was once asked, by a fellow PWP, whether I thought PD had made me a better person, and it was tough to answer. In one sense I'm far more selfish than I was: doing what I want when I want, while I can. I used to prevaricate. I used to not make decisions, especially when it came to things that I considered to be risky, or to be something that might damage my reputation (whatever that is). I would often hedge my bets, try to please both sides. Now, I make decisions. They may often be the wrong ones, and they may often cause me more trouble than I banked on ... but I then deal with the problems as or if and when they occur. My default mode used to be no. Now it's full speed ahead and damn the torpedoes. Selfish, me. The flipside of this is that I do more for others. Again, this may be considered selfish, that I do things to make myself feel good. Well, guilty as charged (though I believe that these things are good in and of themselves, also). This behaviour is good – it's only dubious when it's unacknowledged, when you fail to admit to yourself that this is the way in which you now operate. If you deny that you are behaving in such a manner, it seems to me that you run the risk of according your decisions too much weight, and may fail to reverse or re-assess one of them when you run into trouble.

Compulsive? Moi?

While writing this I'm flicking compulsively backwards and forwards, to and from an internet dating site. It might just as easily be internet shopping or gambling. The kinds of things I hear from other PWP are 'I spend more money than before … but still not as much as my wife, so it's ok'. Dopamine agonists seem to cause a problem with appetites … the 'one just isn't enough' syndrome, whether it's a throw of the dice, a profiterole, or a date. As with hallucinations, reality takes a back seat. There seems to be a connection between dopamine agonists and an inability to say no. An inability to stop. A desire to try just one more. To do it again. To do it again.

It's difficult to divorce this issue from the thorny word 'addict', and I suppose it's accurate, to a degree. It is a highly emotive and, for most, terrifying word. Like the ads on American TV say: denial is the first symptom. Perhaps if I don't deny it, it won't be true.

Ok.

Caveat lector

(That means reader beware, by the way).

Those of you who are judgemental, unsympathetic or generally predisposed towards cynicism, step away from chapter five now. Likewise anyone who knows me, and especially is either related to or has had relations with me. Promise? That's what I want to say. But I'll steam ahead.

Ok. Here goes.

I don't gamble.

It's never been my thing.

I don't compulsively eat.

It's really not my thing (though it's true I suffer a little from the 'just one more ...' syndrome at times).

What I do is fuck. I am, or I became, to all intents and purposes, a sex addict.

And no, that does not meant I needed a fix three times a day, every day. Well, there have been days when I have had sex three times in a day, travelling from (or welcoming in) three different women within twelve hours. Breakfast. Lunch. Dinner. I'm employing purposefully brutal language here. Not because that's how I thought of these women (though if you're someone who ignored my caveat, you may disagree with this estimation), but to ensure that it's practically impossible to identify anyone.

For three years or so, I indulged myself in what many might say was an excessive number of sexual partners, some of whom I also had relationships with. Some of these partners have known that they were not the only individual with whom I was having sexual relations; some (and towards the end of this industrial sowing of oats, hardly any), were not aware. At certain times, I maintained an ever-revolving harem, numbering at its largest seven individuals. As one became disillusioned with my behaviour and decided to move on, I would find another to replace them. During some periods, I would have one lover whom I would treat as if she were exclusive, while indulging myself now and again with others. Sometimes I would go for months with only one partner, sometimes I would barely make two days, or hours, before finding myself swapping one pair of arms for another.

I know I risk alienating you, but I'm simply trying to give you just the tiniest inkling of what it feels like. What it feels like to want to log on one more time, to see whether you can find one more interesting person who might not mind *too* much … how much time I invested in setting up and maintaining different identities on different sites. How difficult it can be to remember what you've said to whom, where they came from initially, how much time it took simply logging on to the different sites to check on the latest round of messages. The endless online chats. How it felt when, on sending a picture to one potential partner, the reply read 'omg. I know you. We can't play.' And no, they didn't reveal themselves. The waiting. The logging back on. The knocking on strange new doors. The endless texts.

I was fortunate, I suppose. Being single (my marriage had broken up before these particular side-effects manifested themselves), I didn't really see it as a compulsion. I was merely doing what every single man does, or wishes he could do (or so I told myself), and what more single women than you may think do. I once went on a date. On the way to her place, she said something like 'is this internet dating just a shagfest, then?' Naturally, I answered in the affirmative.

I would go to a party. I would talk to a girl for ten minutes before saying 'shall we go to my flat and fuck?' and then doing exactly that. I would meet people online, chat for half an hour, be in bed with them twenty minutes later.

I was simply doing what guys do, right? As a teenager I suffered from the common male affliction of not knowing what to do. I never really got involved in the merry-go-round of casual sex. And back then I was always in relationships, and frighteningly jealous and moralistic. Before PD, when presented with no-comeback, no-risk of being caught sexual opportunities I would simply say no (no matter what my loins said). This was perhaps the first thing that changed. I no longer said no.

It took a while before I realised that what was apparently all in fun was actually a compulsion.

Now, as Frank Zappa almost said, was it the drugs, or was it the disease? Well, I'm pretty sure it was a combination of both. Remember that this chapter is ostensibly about making a plan of action. Or perhaps it's more about exploring those things that seem to prevent your making any sort of plan at all. As you yourself may be, I was in an odd situation. Perhaps a rather terrible situation.

I had contracted or developed (I'm not sure how to describe it) an incurable, degenerative brain disease. It meant, oh, I didn't really understand what it meant, but the visions were of a trembling, shuffling, incontinent version of me. I didn't much like this image. My marriage had collapsed under the strain (though there were already problems – perhaps without these we may have survived, perhaps without the Parkinson's we would have split anyway) and I had found myself living in a small room in a town in which almost everyone I knew was from my (impendingly ex) wife's circle. I was lonely and needed some sort of support, no matter how fleeting. So naturally, I went online. Without wanting to sound overly self-absorbed (any more than writing a book about myself and my relationship with a disease already makes me), I'm a reasonably good-looking chap, and I have some ability with words. These are the two things you need online. I got replies. I went on dates. And all the time there were two things running through my head. Well, more than two things, but two important things. The first was that in a few short years I would shuffle to dates, they'd stand up to walk away and I'd piss myself as they did so. Yes, this is a somewhat pessimistic view of things, but that was the future I saw looming ahead of me. There would be no dates. No sex. No love. No support. The second was that as soon as I admitted that I had PD, any possible blooming of romance would simply snuff out.

So when it was offered, I took it. Sex, support, romance, even love. And it was offered a lot, even if these offers took a fairly sizeable investment of time and energy on my part.

You see? Would you think you had a problem? The initial impulse was entirely understandable, a reaction to the state of psychological distress in which I found myself. The continuation was more to do with the drugs.

Reader, things got severely out of hand. I did and said things pre-PD Pete would have simply found unforgivable. People got hurt. One of them was me. Another was a woman with whom I had a relationship for much of this period. I loved her (yes, this capacity remains), and still miss her. The fact that I asked her to edit this book for me shows the respect I have for her: the fact that she agreed is all you need know about her own strength of character.

I have heard other PWP say they are terrified of agonists, and I can understand why. Were I married with a family, this cycle of events would have been simply devastating. It would have ruined lives. I was offered support in the form of a Parkinson's nurse. I simply never got around to it. Another early-onset PWP of my acquaintance (oddly enough, living on the same road as I was at the time when we were both diagnosed) was told there were no other PWP in our area under 50. Typically, we met because I dated a friend of hers, who I met on the internet. So, not all bad, right?

But think very carefully about your therapies, and especially about the drugs. I don't for a moment recommend not taking them (well, some of them, but I suspect that the lawyers might have a dig if I mentioned them by name and why), just that you exercise caution and foresight, and that you gather around yourself as much support as you can. Yes, you can do it alone, but really, don't if you don't have to.

In addition, be warned of one of the other apparent compulsions, but this time, directed at you. If you take the public route in order to raise money and awareness, as I have, albeit on a very low level until now, you will receive messages such as this:

Hi Pete,
sorry to read in the ---- you have Parking disease at such an early age.
I might be able to help cure or at least slow its advance & improve your health
I am a retired pharmacist & have found by a sheer fluke about how most diseases, Arthritis, Diabetes, Heart disease., Cancer, parkinsons etc are caused by acids stored in our bodies by our immune system to prevent it getting into our blood which has an alkaline ph of about 7.4.
Drinking Magnetized water with a ph of 7.7 on an empty

stomach helps detox our body of these acids & eating a less acid diet, avoid fizzy drinks, tea, sugar, coffee. sugar & red meat & eat alkaline dried fruits like Apricots, Figs, Prunes, Raisins as snacks instead of biscuits . might help your condition.

Will forward full details when I have your email address. Its a little known subject & should help.

Now, I have no doubt that this individual was being entirely genuine, and the dietary tips are, by and large, reasonably sound – though, of course, they will doubtless have no particular effect on PD. But for me (and this is me), when I read things like 'magnetized water', I roll my eyes and sigh deeply. Not least because so far as my understanding of magnetism goes, it's pretty much not something you can do to water.

There's a certain breed of people who wish to deny all the advances of western medicine, just as there are those who will countenance no other type of treatment. I'm in no way blind to its faults, but neither am I cynically ruling it out. People are quick to assume 'it's natural so it's good for you/it's a drug therefore it's bad', but I give you digitalis. I give you aspirin. Digitalis is a very potent toxin, as well as being used as a heart medication. Aspirin is a wonderful drug which also can cause haemorrhaging. Both are derived from plants, namely the foxglove and the willow, respectively … it's really about whatever works, whatever you feel comfortable with. PD is incurable. It's caused by the death of brain cells. So far as I'm aware, there is no mechanism that allows them to regenerate. We may discover one. Until then, PD, if it's with you, is with you to stay. There's no point trying to fight it. Accept it, but don't let it rule you. That's my advice.

I have met several people who want to cure me. I'm sure they think they can. I'm equally sure they cannot.

There have been times when I've engaged with people online who blithely state that they have the cure. I have pointed out the truth of the matter that it's incurable, even though there are various therapies which are effective, if only for finite periods, and accompanied by risks and side-effects. The kind of idiotic thing you think might help. Now, I'm happy to agree to disagree, but when one delightful individual decided to tell me it was my attitude which caused it in the first place, let's just say it's lucky that he wasn't saying it to my face, that he chose the relative safety of an internet forum to do so. The anger that wells up inside as a result of this sort of thing is quite astonishing. For this reason I now not only tend to avoid reading much on the internet, let alone commenting, but on those odd occasions when I forget my own rules and get involved, I mostly shut the conversation down pretty sharpish when I get even an inkling that someone is heading in that direction.

This chapter has been hard to write. It was ostensibly about making a plan of action, but it's perhaps obvious that what I've failed to do is make a plan. There is a simple reason for this. The fact is that I do not know what my future holds, and yet I know it all too well. The real problem is the when. I don't know when the PD will be most of me, when to the outside I'll appear as a shuffling set of symptoms. What I've realised is that plans don't really come into it any more. I work much more on a day-by-day basis, reacting to new problems as they turn up. Mostly this is because with such a set of impending issues, it can be easy to be overwhelmed, and worry so much about the future that the present goes begging. I have no idea where I'll be in five years, so why waste energy?

It's difficult not to think bleak thoughts when you have PD. It's difficult not to think that you're fundamentally broken, that either your partner will leave, or if you're single, that no-one in their right mind would connect with you.

This is without doubt overly pessimistic, but there is some truth in it. Finding a balance between pessimism and realism is the most important, and most difficult, thing you'll need to do.

The future is another country, they do things differently there. Do what feels right, surround yourself with as much support as you can. Live. It's what you have now that counts.

A world too wide –
on placing yourself in the scheme of things

Now. Let's not get carried away here. PD isn't the worst thing that can happen. Compared with some conditions and diseases, it's relatively mild. It's not going to kill you in six months. You're not going to lose limbs. It's really not that bad. Is it?

This may seem like a strange way to start a chapter, questioning the seriousness of the disease the whole book's about, but other people will be thinking this; other people will be saying this, if not to you, to others. It's been made a few times to me, the 'it's not so bad', 'you don't look so bad', 'it's only mild, then', the classic 'you wouldn't know' comment, and so on. And they're right. In the grand scheme of things, it's pretty minor. The world is big. There's a lot of stuff in it. An awful lot of it is bad. I've felt guilty for feeling the way I sometimes do about it. Because I know that in many, many ways I'm blessed. And I don't mean that in a tree-hugging, pseudo-spiritual manner, I mean it in simple terms. In terms of plusses and minuses, if you place me (and you, too) on the sliding scale of fortune, well, we're up there. You know we are. This disease in absolute terms is merely an inconvenience. Just a bit of a pain. A progressive, incurable pain, yes, but merely a bit of a pain.

But we don't deal in absolutes. We're not built that way. We're brought up in a society that gives us expectations, and it's those expectations that are stripped from us by this disease. We're surrounded by messages telling us that we can be anything we choose, if only we do x. Of course, we know intellectually that this is nonsense, but the messages are powerful, and powerful messages act powerfully. Furthermore, the advent of a condition such as Parkinson's changes the context of everything that we see, everything that we think, everything that we hope. It robs us of our birthright – at least, what we consider to be our birthright.

I started to see things in terms of negatives. I'd see an advert for something or other with shiny, happy oldies (you know, people 20 years older than me – they're old people) doing shiny, happy things and it was all I could do not to shout out loud that I'd either not make it that far or that I'd be a drooling, shuffling fool by then. I'd receive the annual report on my (rather meagre) private pension, and wonder why I was bothering. (Actually, that's a good point, you'll need to reconsider all your long-term financial plans and expectations, but I'll let you get on with that). I'd see an advert for some geriatric device and I'd try to calculate when I'd need it. I wouldn't make sixty, I wouldn't be able to live in my house in a decade because of the stairs – indeed, I decided against one house because the stairs to the basement kitchen were steep and narrow. Perfect PD accident waiting to happen. Of course, I then put some steep, narrow stairs in my new house. I am, it seems, part denier, part neurotic, part brinksman, part tempter of fate.

I lost my sense of self for a time, and in many ways it was because of the strange status PD affords: cripple-in-waiting. Now, I use such language (and it's my book, so I'll write what I please) entirely knowingly and on purpose. In x years, I will be …

And there's the rub: the integer x. The value of x can only be accurately predicted simultaneously with the outcome '…'.

On letting the world in on the secret

Newly diagnosed, dosed-up and not presenting a wild tremor or any other obvious physical manifestations was, it turned out, a frustrating combination. I wrote an article for the Independent on being diagnosed before I had considered that this was, to all intents and purposes, my 'coming out'. Having since seen how some struggle to go public, I'm glad I did it instinctively, but it has, I believe, had quite a serious effect on my life. On going public I became googleable, and becoming googleable meant that jobs in my particular sphere became even harder, if not impossible, to get. I was told by a colleague that I'd be rejected for most jobs out of hand simply because of the PD. This is, of course, illegal, but no-one, including me, would ever know. And yes, my blog is fuel, too – I noticed that every time an application went in, views went up. It's a problem one might be tempted to conclude was of my own making ... and perhaps I was 'asking for it' by talking openly about my condition.

This particular problem opened up a whole new way of thinking for me. Suddenly I was looking at the 'disabled' section and wondering whether I ought declare myself as such. But this was fraught with contradictions, not least the fact that I was not, and am not, disabled, nor do I consider myself to be. I don't receive disability benefits (unlike some PWP, who both need and deserve such benefits), because I haven't applied for them (I wouldn't get them anyway. Because I'm not disabled). Right now I'm what might reasonably be termed 'directly inconvenienced', I suppose. In some senses, quite markedly.

I have a three-year driving licence, which naturally doesn't make me feel great about myself, but I'm not disabled. And yet it appears that I'm discriminated against on the grounds that I am. Which means that I am disabled. By people's attitudes. Because of the drugs I take, I can't even be that sure how I'd be sans medication ... a state that might perhaps be a decent indicator of status.

I occupy a grey area, a simultaneous state of disabled/not disabled. In this zero sum game I am both 0 and 1. I am Parkinson's Cat, my superposition of states collapsed only by the introduction of the integer x, which itself simultaneously represents a numeral relating to my post-diagnostic age (I am four and a half), a particular task or physical operation, or perhaps an algorithm. Cathy added that this was 'probably the most unreadable sentence I've had the pleasure of this week', which is about right, because unreadable is how I feel half the time.

I am me but not me. And it is in this state that we are forced to search for a place to inhabit, a position to adopt, a lifestyle to choose, while all around the hawkers and snake-oil salesmen jabber in our ears, trying to catch the last vestiges of our hope on their cunning little hooks.

In many ways, I was knocked off-centre by my diagnosis. It left me unbalanced, insecure, unconvinced. I was unbalanced because there was something else forming the being I liked to call me. Something over which I had no control. PD snuck in through the back door. One day, on arriving home, I found it ensconced in the sitting room, occupying my favourite chair and warming its toes by the fire. This unbalancing naturally affects everyone around you, and the closer they are, the greater the effect. It is an unsettling feeling, the renegotiation of the self, but this is exactly what needs to occur. The economist John Maynard Keynes once said: 'When the facts change, I change my mind: what, Sir, do you do?' On diagnosis, the facts well and truly change. In the seventeenth century, a 'fact' was a piece of information that was to be proven or disproven in court. The fact was the thing, the crime, the action, the happening, accusation: the court was to decide on its truth and relevance. This is just like diagnosis – the fact is the diagnosis, and it seeks approval in the MRI scans, the DAT scans, the levodopa challenge, the twisting of the wrist, the writing, the walking. On diagnosis, the facts about the self (all held rather inconveniently by the self) all change, and the self must be re-negotiated: the life re-examined, the new facts incorporated into the new self. This new self invariably needs help.

Its security rocked by the information implicit within the diagnosis, the new self lacks several luxuries afforded the old self. And the more it (the self) tries to learn about what this diagnosis entails, in the hope of re-asserting (self) control, the more shaky things become. It's a strange process in which an increase in knowledge leads to a decrease in certainty. The more you learn about what PD does, how it progresses and how it affects people differently, the more unsure the future becomes.

Below are the reactions I have recognised. They are in no particular order, because I do not wish to imply that there are specific stages that one necessarily goes through, or that the reaching of a particular stage is to be desired or aimed for:

Calm acceptance
Stoicism
Rage
Denial
Embracing
Resistance
Active fighting

These reactions all manifest in different people in different ways. I have been through several of them, often more than one simultaneously. I have flitted between them. I have denied, like my Biblical namesake, that I can even be said to have adhered to any of them in particular. And yet I can go from raging against the injustice of it all to simply shrugging my shoulders and intoning 'whatever' in the blink of an eye.

In the meantime, I have been subjected to countless diatribes concerning how I 'ought' to react to having this disease. There are innumerable books and self-help courses available that chart an almost Buddhist path for you through life and through various traumas, stating clearly and confidently that you must do x, then y will follow, and eventually you will arrive at z – and these books and courses are distilled and poured into my ears by innumerable well-meaning individuals. The journey metaphor, as a good friend suggested to me when I began to write this book, has pretty much been done. To death, one might say, but we'll come back to that one. This prescriptive way of viewing things is, to my mind, fraught with danger, as without a whole bucketload of self-delusion we're never going to go though our life making smooth transitions from one stage to the next.

I know I have imposed a seven-stage map on this book, but as you'll have noticed by now, the actual progression, like that of a life, is very different. It's messy, jerky, blurred round the edges and misty in the middle. It's snakes and ladders crossed with Cluedo superimposed onto Mousetrap with a hint of Operation!, all played in the dark, on a pitching boat, while wearing boxing gloves smeared with Vaseline. Each stage has substages, and each substage yet further substages, ad infinitum. It's a little like Zeno's paradox concerning Achilles and the Tortoise, which suggests that Achilles may catch up, but can never overtake, the tortoise. Except that we always, but always, are overtaken.

To me, however, it's actually quite simple.

If you want to rage against the injustice of it all, howl at the moon and tear at your breast with your nails, then knock yourself out. It won't do any good, but it may make you feel better.

If you want to bury your head in the sand, hide behind the sofa with your fingers over your eyes, then knock yourself out. It won't do any good, but it may make you feel better.

If you want to come out fighting, show this bastard disease what's what, then knock yourself out. It won't do any good, but it may make you feel better. And so on.

It seems to me that trying to do something that doesn't fit with your character is fraught with difficulties. My self was rocked quite enough by Dr Parkinson's shaking palsy when it took up residence, and I think that wildly changing my world view in response to it would simply have made things even worse. As it was, my marriage dissolved, my career took a nose-dive, my behaviour changed and my future became shorter and less pleasant. There wasn't a lot left to hold on to. I did, however, finally have some sort of explanation for those little things that were going wrong. I knew that I wasn't being neurotic, that I wasn't being hypochondriac, that I wasn't denying that the inevitable (ageing) happens.

There is a balance to be had. Everyone will tell you that you mustn't become defined by your disease, that you must hold on to your youness, and yet, part of that you is now the disease. You can't hold on to your youness without Parky becoming at least part of the you that you want to keep. It's a bugger, but it's *our* bugger. As my condition has progressed, I've found that I spend increasing amounts of time doing things to take the edge off the symptoms, avoiding things that remind me what I've got, or dealing with what it throws at me today. The fact is that this disease takes over your life, slowly but surely, invading every part of your body and doing funny things to your head.

Yes, you need to watch your diet, and yes, you need to exercise, and yes, you need to be more careful, generally, when it comes to many things, but most importantly, you need to listen. Listen to what your body and your brain are saying. I know it sounds poncy, but it's so easy to get lost, to get swept away by the tidal wave of despair, anger, confusion, that you need to anchor yourself somewhere, and that somewhere is you. You need to retain as much self-awareness as possible, because you're truly all you have to rely on. All the PD support groups, the friends, relatives, lovers, partners, not one of them can do a damn thing to help unless they know what is going on. I sent the first four chapters of this book to several people, including one of my sisters. She wrote the following:

"Just read first two chapters ... I can't say I am enjoying it, well perhaps I can because it is fluent, informative and not patronising (at least I don't feel that it is). The bit I am not enjoying is the squirming feeling it is leaving me with as I am forced to confront the extent to which I have abandoned my little brother to himself without ever pausing to listen."

Now, that may seem like an odd thing to quote here, perhaps even a little self-serving, but it's the second sentence that confuses me. It confuses me because I simply don't recognise this abandonment, or this lack of listening. The truth of the matter is that I have not said much that might have been listened to and no-one's been given the chance to abandon me, as I've pretty much hermetically sealed myself off from all and sundry other than in my blog. It's all down to how you react as an individual, how much you tell people about how you're feeling about the whole, sorry mess. There have been moments when I have.

When my father was in the last few weeks of his life, in the last stages of acute myeloid leukaemia, we agreed a sort of unspoken truce between us. The antagonism we had shared for so many years seemed all rather pointless, rather self-indulgent, so we shelved it. He did, at one point, say 'I never did understand why we didn't get on', and it seemed rather gauche to point out the many, many reasons beyond the stark-staringly obvious one. So, uncharacteristically, I held my tongue. Years before, we had been in the middle of some pointless argument when I said: 'You know what your trouble is? You're just like your father.' To which he (reasonably) replied 'and doesn't that mean you're just like me?' A good point. 'Yes', I said. 'The difference is I know it.'

It may seem odd that he keeps turning up in these pages, but actually it makes perfect sense. I am more like him than I perhaps care to admit, and while his life's trajectory was very different to mine, he, like me (or me, like he) was struck down by a condition that in itself was not fatal, merely debilitating, but which led to things that are dangerous to life and limb. He always said that he wouldn't make old bones, and he was absolutely correct. Odd that he understood this, as one of his many problems was an acute lack of self-awareness. Or, possibly, an inability to act upon or cope with the self-awareness he did possess.

Having registered his confusion at our apparently incomprehensible and lifelong clashing of horns, he then followed it up with 'and if you think I was bad, you should have met my father'. A strange thing to say, as I did meet, and know, his father, my grandfather. He was an irascible, unpleasant man, who did strange things. He would, for example, throw the picnic lunch you brought when visiting him away, so that when you opened the fridge, there was nothing there. A moment's confusion followed by the realisation that opening the bin would reveal all. Once, when I was staying with my grandparents at an age tender enough that I needed the landing light left on, he convinced me that the bulb that died during the night was one that had been performing landing duties for thirty years, ladling the guilt on with a long-handled spoon.

Impending death brought a clarity to my father's thoughts, albeit with regards what might be considered mere trifles, such as wine. That particular conversation went something like this (and I'm not even attempting to capture his voice, as it's so similar to mine that I am utterly incapable of hearing it):

D: You know what's really annoying?

P: No, obviously not.

D: Hmph. Well, a few years ago I bought a load of wine so that I might have some good claret in my dotage, and now I'm not going to be able to enjoy it.

P: Well, there's a simple solution! Get drinking before it's too late … after all, it's not like it's going to damage your health or anything.

D: Yes, you'd think. But whether it's the disease or the chemo, I don't know, but I simply can't stand the taste.

Before any family meal, he'd open a bottle, let it breathe for a few hours, take a sip, try not to gag, and watch us enjoy it.

What he had done was perfectly reasonable. He had planned for what he expected would happen. For what ought to have happened. For what was most likely to happen. He wasn't to know that the expected was going to be headed off at the pass by some bastard disease, albeit one for which a cure is possible. The unexpected, the unknown, is always something of a surprise, by definition. It's perhaps counter-intuitive to suggest this, but the expected, the known, is sometimes more shocking. It's the when that gives the expected its great power. The monster in the horror movie that you know is waiting. When you turn the corner and it's *this* corner around which a particular unpleasantry lies, the shock is all the more poignant because you ought to have seen it coming. Naturally, this ignores the fact that it's a) waiting and b) hiding around the corner.

Each corner has another quality, of course; that of invisibility. We walk on in what appears to be a straight line and yet we are constantly beset and besieged, ambushed by our bodies and our minds as each corner is unknowingly turned. People often bring up the 'but you could get hit by a bus tomorrow' line when I suggest that the mindset of the PWP is different to theirs because of the certain knowledge of the uncertainty which awaits. My usual retort is that the PWP is hit by a bus every fucking day. And it takes its toll.

On the subject of walking, one night a friend asked me why I was walking with a limp. This was because my left heel was brushing the ground with every step. It's known as the Parkinson's shuffle: the gait becomes more compromised, and the strides become shorter as the body stiffens. I can walk normally, but I have to concentrate to make it happen, I have to actively do what my body now refuses to do instinctively. I know that the problem is simply that my left foot refuses to acknowledge the position of the ground, but it's been, up until now, something that few people have noticed. It troubles me, but I am aware that this disease makes me hyper-sensitive with regards changes in my physical being. Well, perhaps hyper-neurotic might be more accurate, but this neurosis doesn't necessarily mean the things that I notice are irrelevant. I have lost count of the number of times that, on describing some of the effects of PD in the wider sense, the stiffness, the slowness, the simple grinding inefficiency of your body when in its thrall, I've met with an indulgent look and a 'we're all getting old, pal'. But that's the point. I regularly have trouble getting out of bed. I stumble, I shuffle, I make the noises my father made on getting up out of a chair … when he was in his sixties. Yes, some of the symptoms of PD are remarkably like ageing. But, get this: we're not all fucking old!

To heap insult onto brain injury, the whole process is so utterly random as to be completely unpredictable. I have no clue from one day to the next just how my body's going to behave. What I do know is that while I seem to have no direct way of improving matters – it simply does what it wishes to do when it so desires – I can make things worse. I can make them worse by being inactive, by refusing to do the things that PD makes difficult, by giving in to the disease.

I know I cannot win. I know that there is no way to fight it. I also know that the less I do, the quicker the corners come around, the faster the progression. I know this from spending seven weeks in a sling following the operation on my shoulder. By the time I could release my arm, my left hand was barely able to move. But for all that I know this to be true, there's no substitute for seeing it. Sometimes when you see yourself, you see someone else. It's your old self looking at your new self: your now self looking at your soon self.

Here's a blog post I wrote after one such moment, when the two selves caught up with one another.

Serendipitiful [first published 6 Sept 2012]

It is often said that the best way of finding something is by not looking for it, and goodness I found something yesterday. By accident. En passant. While searching for the answer to something else.

I took my trusty camerawoman to a weekday game at Streat and Westmeston Cricket Club, a beautiful little ground nestling in the grounds of Middleton Manor, just outside Ditchling. From the pavilion the views of the Downs and the Beacon are truly beautiful, and the day could not have been a better one: a sharp contrast to last week's drizzly affair at Sidley, near Bexhill. The camera was there for a clear purpose: to allow me to talk a little about my preparation and how I feel about playing, in the hope that I, or someone, might come up with some ideas about how to mend my head.

I am, you see, increasingly coming to believe that my game is now played out in the head. Yes, I have technical faults, but these are minor. I'm trying to bridge the gap between practice and performance. In training I am positive, decisive, effective. In the middle I am, at present at least, all at sea. And generally out for a teeny weeny score.

So. Video. Can I see things which I might accentuate or minimise in order to play some decent cricket?

What I saw was actually quite shocking. I walk like an old person.

Over the past year, I've gone from being co-ordinated and fluid in my movements to being stiff, jerky and shuffling.

Now, when I walk, my torso is stiff and upright, my stride short, my legs moving as if I'm protecting my knees, or at least have very solid knee braces on. My arms, and especially my left arm, barely swing at all, my shoulders are stiff and solid, with none of the rolling movement one sees in the, oh fuck … I've backed myself into a corner … healthy.

I am ill.

Yesterday I seriously considered stopping playing. I'm simply not convinced I can take the humiliation for much longer.

Just as I watch myself on video, and see myself stiff, upright, left arm clamped by my side, so I am sometimes confronted with myself in others. My brother-in-law sent me a link to a short piece on a baseball player, Ben Petrick, who was diagnosed at 23. I recognised much of what he talked about, and he even did the finger-waggling comparison I do. But he had one thing that I managed to escape: his life was, it seemed, effectively ruined. He ploughed on playing baseball for another three years but he gradually deteriorated to the point where it was becoming noticeable. I thought about this process about six months after my diagnosis. I considered just how devastated I would have felt if I were still a professional musician. I would have watched my living, my reason for living, my way of earning a living, simply waste away. I would have done the same as Petrick, and hidden my disease, despaired as my talent slowly ebbed away. Instead, I was, in some ways, lucky. When PD arrived, it arrived in a body that was not particularly vital to the carrying out of my life. While yes, I was very physical and physically fit, it was because I liked to be, not because I had to be. I paid attention to my physicality because I wanted to, because it gave me, it gives me, something on which to focus my attention, something I can measure myself with – even if what I'm measuring is my downfall.

My reaction to all of this nonsense, this gradual but consistent deterioration, has been mixed, and twofold. I work increasingly on my physical fitness and co-ordination. As my winter's lay-off from the gym and other things has shown me (if, indeed, I needed to be shown), the less active you are, the more unable you become. It's not, it seems, that exercise arrests the decline, merely that it makes the decline less apparent. As well as the problems with walking, with my left hand, with my co-ordination, with the general speed of my body's movements, with the stiffening of the tendons, PD also slowly destroys the musculature. Muscles do a lot more than allow us to lift things. They work in concert, a series of elastic bands all balanced and taut, keeping things together and fluid. You walk from the legs upwards, from the shoulders downwards, through the hips. Keeping them in good shape helps hold the body together. Letting them atrophy allows those things that knock us off balance – right-handedness, injury, Parkinson's – to take over and skew and twist and mess us up. What happens next is simple. Things become increasingly difficult to do, so we stop doing them. This leads to their becoming increasingly difficult to do.

There is no magic solution. There is no one approach that works. Anything you do helps ... anything. I work out at the gym, I play cricket, I will soon re-commence training in one or another martial art (though one less likely to break me than before), and I dance. But it's difficult. It's difficult because no matter how hard you train, you still go backwards. The training merely helps slow the rate down. It's difficult because there are always days when the PD beats you all ends up, when no matter what you try, you simply can't.

These days are simply the most depressing, when you're working all out to make your world at least a little more bearable, and it is taken well and truly out of your hands. And yet from these moments new hope can spring, new desire can form. It's a question, for me at least, not of fighting or resisting or of not going gently into that good night, but of simply saying well, OK, that's fucked – how can I fix it? And if you can't, well, then it's time to make a quick analysis. When I had my shoulder operation in December, I knew full well that I would not have a fully functioning left arm until the end of May, a good six weeks into the cricket season. I was left with a stark choice: bat left-handed, or simply don't play. Cricket for me is therapy, and while I'm not exactly the most competent player, it's something I enjoy. The problems I've been having with my left hand have had an impact on my game, as I regularly lose grip of the bat, playing false shots as I do so. My decision to bat left-handed gave me a no-pressure opportunity to experiment, to play without my dodgy hand. Because the chances were I'd have to change eventually anyway. Then, as the season went on and my shoulder healed, I refused to give in, no matter how depressing my season's run tally became. Bloody-mindedness that is in many ways counter-productive, but allows me to feel real.

This reality gave me a unique opportunity to help other PWP by getting sponsorship for every run I scored. This, again, is something I see a lot – the urge in the PWP to enumerate the experience, to make a tangible contribution, a contribution that can be measured, that can be recorded. Why? I'm not entirely sure, but it may be something to do with the way in which PD is so subjective and changeable, so personal, that to submit it to some sort of measurement just feels good. There, I did £65 of helping PWP today, I would say as I left the crease. It also helped me feel better about my supposed failures ... if I turned it into cash, it seemed a lot more useful.

My aim was to use the money to set up a tango workshop for PWP, primarily because tango is at heart an assisted walk with an added hug – and that can only be a good thing. This may sound overly reductive – a walking hug – but sometimes that's really the only way to look at things. Parkinson's, like many other conditions, can easily lead you down a vicious spiral from which it is extremely hard to escape. The depression you can feel on being diagnosed, that feeling that life is over, can easily drift into an inability to do anything, aided and abetted by the depression the PD can cause rather more chemically. It may start by your simply feeling down, but soon you have the means of getting up again taken away. Add this to the possibility that your behaviour might be contributing to your mood, and things stand a good chance of drifting out of arm's reach. I have noticed this in myself from time to time. This blog post considers a time when external factors caused by my behaviour collided with internal imbalances, when some of my actions came back to haunt me, and combined perfectly with the changes in my brain chemistry to create misery.

Slings and Arrows [first published 6 Dec 2011]

The last few days have been troubling for me. There are various events that I could point to, various people who, wittingly or not, have added to the sea of troubles against which I must choose to set myself against or drown, a peasant of infinite space. But I shall not. Point, that is. I was told from an early age that it was rude to do so, even though this virtual world invites if not actively encourages it. I have been pointed at, and I have been traduced in forums where I could, had I wished to, retort in like manner. I chose not to, and still do so, I expect that any right-thinking person will recognise the signs of a partial account and dismiss these from their view. Likewise, when bile of any sort is spewed. Those who cannot see past the darkly sparkly bits? Well, I care not for them nor their opinions.

But the troubles which beset me are wider and deeper than the bleatings of a few. One of the things about PD that I sometimes forget was pointed out to me by my neurologist yesterday. While discussing the gradual decline in motor function, and the increasing vulnerability to physical injury to which I find myself prone, the topic of mood came up. He noted that while the obvious symptoms were physical, the gradually worsening gait, the loss of fine motor control, the gentle introduction of what will be my tremor, and all the rest of it, it must be remembered that PD is a neurological disorder. It is your brain fucking up. The sloshing chemical soup of your grey matter is changing, adjusting, and certain chemicals, namely dopamine, are becoming more and more rare. This leads to more than simply physical symptoms.

Reader, I'm depressed.

Not terribly, but enough to know that it's more than simply feeling a little glum. I struggle to motivate myself to do most anything: even getting out of bed is becoming a little bit of a chore. I can barely place one creative word in the wake of another.

Now, PD is not something which lends itself to bouts of cheery optimism. After all, you see and feel your body crumble day by day. You walk up the road and you are convinced that everyone looking at you wonders why you're drunk so early in the morning. You look forward not to a happy, healthy future, but one in which your physical self is gradually ground down, your personality squashed.

You become your illness. Not just to others, but to yourself.

It's not simply that PD is a depressing thing to have, but that it can lead to depression itself, and a depression which sits, fat and heavy, upon your chest. Almost as if you're being pressed … an old technique for proving testimony. If you insisted on sticking by your story when your ribs were cracking, then it seemed reasonable to think that you were being honest.

I see many things which weigh upon me. People with academic jobs with no publications. People who know how to sell themselves. People who play a role so perfectly. People who seem to hold cards I do not. People who paint me the villain when villain I am not.

These are the things which flatten, which allow the claws to get into my flesh, to hold me to the floor while the world seems to pile its weight upon me. I will not retract, so on the piling goes, and deeper the claws pierce.

If the disease can lead to bouts of depression, then the drugs themselves have their own problems. I am on Mirapexin, or pramipexole, a dopamine agonist. It is designed to stimulate the cells whose job it is to produce dopamine, the neural transmitter, to produce more. These are the cells in the basal ganglia which are dying. It's like whipping a dying donkey. It works for a while. This drug has some weird and wonderful side-effects. I used to hallucinate regularly, especially with regards rushing, scuttling things in my peripheral vision, and mislabelling normal phenomena — seeing a spider scuttle to and fro instead of the shadow of the bathroom light cord.

Another side-effect, and here it's drug and disease colluding in a ludicrous way, is that I combine obsessive compulsive behaviour with an inability to focus. I get lost in the internet, and yet produce nothing. There are other problems with the drug which again combine with the disease to create situations which lead to nothing but trouble.

These problems, and the behaviour to which they led, are contributory factors to the troubles with which I find myself beset. The troubles which feed my depression. It is a vicious, internal circle.

I am ill. This is not an excuse, but a factor which needs to be taken into account.

I need help. I think I'm ready for it now.

A similar thing can happen physically, when inactivity brought on by a feeling that it's all a waste of time seems to allow the disease to take control of your body rather more comprehensively than you might have expected. For me, seven weeks in a sling meant I could barely move my left hand, let alone do stuff. The tremor began then, too, and when I noticed it (it is still erratic) my heart sank. After all, there are milestones in every condition, even when that condition is simply living. My tremor is stress and tiredness related. Nervousness also sets my hand off (though, perhaps oddly, it's my right hand that suffers most). Lack of exercise equals advancing PD equals mild depression equals lack of desire to exercise leads to the whole sorry unmerry-go-round starting again. For an active man whose gym habit began some fifteen years ago, it came as a surprise that it took six months to get back into my stride. Imagine how difficult it would have been to start from new, putting an increasingly truculent body into situations where it simply wants to sulk in the corner.

Tango is something that, for me, is rather useful. It allows the PWP to walk without fear, as they're supported by their partner as a matter of course. It provides social stimulus when the desire to venture outdoors begins to dissipate. It allows you to touch another human without feeling strange or patronised. It helps to make you feel human once more.

There are many activities trumpeted as particularly good for PWP, and while some may well be better than others, to me it doesn't much matter what you're doing as long as you are.

As for finding a place in the scheme of things, this whole sorry saga has made me simultaneously more selfish and more generous. I now do what I want, when I want. Within reason, anyway. I don't understand waiting. I can't plan my next five years because I simply have no idea. Ironically, though, while I was mildly (and not unpleasantly) lost five years ago, the PD that is slowly robbing me of my physicality and various aspects of my personality, and changing my voice for good measure, has actually given me some focus, a compass bearing on which I can direct my energy. I have little choice, as I either roll over and submit or I use it.

Sans everything –
on the unknown

PD is a disease of possibilities. A disease of inevitabilities. A disease of maybes. A disease that goes, like the song, perhaps, perhaps, perhaps. I'm sitting in my office, and typing mostly one-fingered (unless you count my thumb). My mouth is continually filling with saliva, and I choke repeatedly. Only mildly, but choke I do. This happens sometimes, because my swallow reflex goes awol. I know many of the things that might happen to me over the next few years, and I also know some of the things that will happen, because they're already happening. I know that my gait will get worse, my spatial ability will decrease, I'll bump into things, drop things, have difficulty drinking coffee, pints of beer. I'll be treated like I'm drunk when I'm sober, I'll start to lose all the things that make me me.

The fact is that I know *what*, I just don't know *when* (or, in some cases, whether). PD is a gradually debilitating condition. My body will gradually crumble about my brain as I get older. I will watch as I become increasingly unable to carry out those tasks I, even now, find utterly commonplace. What will happen is that my actual and my expected physical condition will become increasingly estranged – two diverging pathways, yet still visible from each other, if only for a while. I will suffer a cartesian version of cognitive dissonance – that is, my mind will know what a healthy body should be capable of, while entombed in an increasingly debilitated one. I've always thought that the very worst part of Alzheimer's must be the possibility that you actually know what's going on. My grandmother was known, in her final, rather difficult weeks, to stop, look my mother in the eye, and say clearly and confidently, 'I do know, you know'. Then she would return to her strange little planet, which to all intents and purposes was, or at least appeared to be, one bereft of any self-awareness, let alone consciousness.

The statistics for PD are less than helpful, not least because they are rather vague when it comes to early onset. If, at diagnosis, you are the more typical age, which is around sixty-three years old, then life expectancy is around fifteen years. This isn't that different from what one might expect anyway, but it's the quality of life rather than the quantity that is at stake. The PWP has an increased risk of developing dementia and depression to add to the physical issues – the falls, the urinary tract infections, the various motor issues. For those diagnosed in their sixties, the disease is very similar to simple old age, with added complications, but an old age that trots ahead somewhat faster than might be considered polite.

If, however, you are diagnosed at or before fifty or even forty years old, then the story is more complicated. The statistics are variable, with some studies suggesting that an early diagnosis can shave up to ten years off life expectancy. Again, the problem is twofold. Firstly, it depends which set of figures you see first, which (let's face it) depends on what website you look at. Different sites suggest different numbers, but then, plus ça change. Secondly, it's the quality of life issue. Early onset patients do tend to progress more slowly than others, but there's some issue separating the disease from regular ageing: when both have similar effects, the cause is more difficult to ascertain but it boils down to further, and faster.

In the early-onset patient, the progression may be slow, but the place it takes you relative to your expectation of ageing is perhaps further, and faster.

Further, and faster. This is what confronted me when I watched my father die at the age of sixty-seven. I saw the moment when what was his consciousness left his body. I have no doubt whatsoever of this. One moment he was a living, feeling being, and one in quite plainly phenomenal quantities of pain, and the next there was simply a body doing what it had to do: anything to stay functioning. The body continued some time after the man had gone. This was not pleasant for any one of us. Why? Because we knew that 'he' was gone, and yet we sat with the machinery waiting for the clockwork to wind down. And we knew that's what we were doing.

Now, until that point of departure, he was plainly suffering. This, again, was not a surprise, and would not have been to him: he was a GP, and would have known exactly what was waiting for him. I still fail completely to understand his thought patterns here.

Why, oh why, did he not end his life when he had the chance? Or, perhaps a more difficult decision, why did he not ask to be palliated to such a degree that his exit was gentle rather than wracked with pain? He had the wherewithal.

I have pondered this question at length. I have yet to come up with a coherent response. I have several ideas, but none of them equates with the man I knew. I mention this because I know, or at least suspect, that at some point I will become something I cannot stand to be. At some point I will be unable to live with myself. This may sound unbearably defeatist, unfeasibly negative, but it is, I think, anything but. I can think of nothing worse or more negative than failing to grasp this particular nettle and finally having my choice in these matters removed.

This matter of freedom of choice is, I believe, utterly paramount. As soon as we blindly give in to anything or adhere to any structure imposed upon us without considering it fully we are reduced, we become lesser beings. The discretion to act as we see fit is paramount – even if in doing so we risk the censure of the society whose rules we must necessarily accept as they are enforced, whether or not we choose to adhere to them. Freedom only works within measurable parameters. As this disease progresses (a progression over which I have no choice), things will slowly be decided for me. My freedom will gradually be whittled away. I will, like a friend also with PD, be forced to accept that I can, or should, no longer play cricket. A tiny, insignificant thing in itself, but indicative of the gradual change in physical circumstances taking over, making my decisions for me. All physical activity will eventually become out of bounds, beyond the pale. I'm worried about writing, especially. My typing has never been the best, but it's getting worse. I can still type at a pace that works for me and my thought processes, but what about when I can't keep up? Well, voice-recognition software, of course. But that, I suspect, will be problematic. My voice is bound to change. Writing and speaking are very different activities indeed. Will I be able to call myself a writer? Will I be able to write at all? Whatever happens, I'll deal with it, but it's something, another thing, over which I will have no choice.

There will come a time when I have no choice left, when I have no ability to direct my life, when I am simply someone for someone else to look after. This I feel may be too much for me to cope with. A friend once said that maybe I ought to cross that bridge when I come to it. I replied that the problem is simply that when I get to that particular bridge, I'll no longer be able to cross it unassisted.

Yes, we're talking euthanasia. This issue crops up periodically in the press, and there was a particular flood of stories after Terry Pratchett went public on being diagnosed as having Alzheimer's, and subsequently took the bull by the horns in the form of a documentary concerning some who had chosen to end their lives. This was immediately leapt upon by an organisation called 'Care, not Killing', a group who, well … let's simply say I disagree most strongly with their beliefs. I disagree most strongly with their beliefs regarding the freedoms one ought to be allowed to enjoy. I disagree most strongly with the manner in which they choose to deny an individual their dignity/ Naturally, I wrote about it.

Care, not killing? Behave … [first published 3 April 2011]

An article in the Guardian this morning, http://www.guardian.co.uk/society/2011/apr/0 3/assisted-dying-nan-maitland-dignitas-arthritis discusses the rather thorny issue of assisted suicide. The particular subject is that of Nan Maitland who, suffering from what she herself described as crippling arthritis, chose, at the age of 84, to end her life at the Dignitas clinic in Switzerland.

As ever, this has proved to be the seat of some controversy, with some suggesting that where the patient does not suffer from a terminal disease, there perhaps ought not be the option of ending one's own life. The article writes that

'Care Not Killing, an alliance that campaigns against assisted dying, said the case demonstrated "a shifting of the goalposts" by pro-rights campaigners and would place pressure on vulnerable people to end their lives if they felt they were a burden. "It's a very scary situation that not very severely disabled people could, at the drop of a hat, opt to kill themselves, and [Maitland's case] shows a ramping-up by campaigners," said a spokesman. "Many people have to live with arthritis. It does expose the lie that only people who are terminally ill will be affected by changes in the law."'

Care not Killing puts me in mind of those delightful American groups which deny the right of a woman to chose to have an abortion, even in the case of rape or incest. Those groups who see no conflict in calling themselves 'pro-life' and murdering doctors who perform such operations. The fact is that anyone can opt to kill themselves 'at the drop of a hat' (wilfully misleading and emotive language if ever I read any — and utterly irresponsible, too) it is only those severely disabled who need assistance. It seems, however, the height of arrogance to insist that those who can, do it themselves (which is the implication of CNK's position), not least as a botched attempt can lead to an agonising death which serves no-one.

It seems to me that Nan Maitland got it right in this instance when she wrote the following:

"For some time, my life has consisted of more pain than pleasure. I have a great feeling of relief that I will have no further need to struggle through each day.

She added: "I have had a wonderful life, and the great good fortune to die at a time of my choosing."

Our lives are our own, and our own to choose to end should we so desire. It's true that a mistaken suicide is not a mistake one learns from, but equally it is not a mistake one lives to regret. Naturally, if one is religious or has belief in a higher being then the argument changes. I do not believe that pressure groups have any right to tell me or anyone how they should live their life — or how, when and why they should end it.

The understanding missing from the arguments of CNK and their ilk is firstly that we will all die — in this respect, arguing that someone is not suffering from an officially terminal disease is somewhat mealy mouthed — and secondly that the only person fit to make a decision regarding the worth of an individual life is the individual themselves. Since my diagnosis, I have considered it a possibility that, at some point, I will choose to end my life before, in the rather intelligent and considered words of Nan Maitland, it consists of considerably more pain than pleasure. And yes, I am aware that Parkinson's is not an especially painful disease. There is more than one type of pain, however.

As I have written before, my particular symptoms are mild enough to go unnoticed by most, though the observant may clock my cack-handedness with forks, for example, and perhaps spot the tremor which has begun to appear at certain times — times of stress and extreme physical tiredness. The lack of pronounced tremor means that the changes I feel within myself are only apparent when expressed. The difficulty swallowing, the increased muscular stiffness which, in turn, has led to an increased propensity to injury … which leads to an inability to train properly, which leads to an increased propensity to injury …

None of these really matter that much, but the fact of the matter is that at some point, I will become unable to do those things which I identify as forming me. I am slowly being robbed of my identity. My brain has increasing difficulty relating to my body. More and more it sees it not as an intrinsic part of 'me', but as a rather recalcitrant and flawed host. A hindrance, not a help.

At some point, I may find that my body and my brain are at such loggerheads that they need to be separated. CNK will presumably want me stuck in a home, a force-fed, arse-wiped, useless body sat staring into the distance, drooling.

This tells me one thing, and one thing only. Groups such as Care not Killing do not understand what life truly is, what makes it such a wonderful, beautiful thing. In failing to accept that it must end, and that we can have control over this end, they turn life into mere mechanics. They truly are fools.

It can be a painful thing to hear, that a loved one is considering ending their own life. When I first began to turn this over in my mind that is exactly what I did: turn it over in my mind. I didn't discuss it with anyone, I didn't seek advice, solace, a second opinion. I did what has become habitual for me: I wrote about it. As has also become common, those people I ought to have talked to found out by reading about it. Much like they will have done while reading this book. When Cathy edited this book, she commented at length on this section, and her comments caused me to rethink my rather defensive tone. I thought it best to simply quote her in full:

> "The first time I saw or heard you mention suicide, we had recently got back together. You wrote it on your blog (heh, because why bother *talking* to me about anything that actually mattered, anyway) and it felt like your words had jumped out of the page and strangled my heart. (Ah yes, here it is on the next page.) Stop spitting, I haven't finished. BUT. That was my first reaction. Shock, horror. And then I thought. And I read. And I raised the topic with you. And I thought some more. And then I thought, and I still think, that I would be there, if you wanted me. Regardless of our relationship and whether it would last, I would not let you make that journey to Switzerland alone (for that is what you were writing about) – unless you expressly wanted to. I ran it through my brain, looked at websites, spent time with myself working out whether I was strong enough. I was, and I am, and if that is what you choose to do, at some hopefully very distant time, you will not go alone unless you wish to."

It's really rather humbling to know that you have such support. More than this, it's really, really good. The only fly in the ointment is that I wonder what the fuck I was playing at, keeping it all to myself, holding it in. Suffering in silence.

And finally

This book is finished, bar the shouting, and for me, the process of looking back has been extremely interesting. It does not, however, compete with the here and now. When this stuff is directly in front of me it can be so clear as to be frightening: it's opacity no less so.

I see myself in others; I see others in myself. I know others with PD and I know that their symptoms lessen in my presence, and this happens in reverse, too. A recent discussion on this subject concluded that – considering stress seems to work to accentuate the visible symptoms of PD – there is a certain lessening of stress due to the fact that you know that the person you are with does more than merely empathises, more than merely understands; they *know*.

This, I believe, is what helps more than anything. It's not the act of talking with someone who knows what it's like (though that in itself is a quite wonderful thing), it's simply feeling that you're not alone. Because if there's one thing I've felt consistently since the very moment of my diagnosis, it's alone. What Cathy wrote in her notes to this final chapter was quite a wake-up call for me. All that time I'd spent feeling alone when all I needed to do was to talk. All I needed to do was to let people in. But PD made me feel so isolated, I was convinced that no-one else could possibly understand. And of that I'm right, but the disease is one thing, the way it affects you is another. PD brings a lot of big issues into focus, and it's these issues which your support network can truly help with. Let them.

If there's one reason why I've written this book, it's so that other PWP, and especially those newly diagnosed, their friends and family, know that they're not alone.

On the author

Writer, academic, cricketer, and musician, Pete Langman lives and works in Brighton.

For more information on Parkinson's disease, these are a very good place to begin:

http://www.parkinsons.org.uk
http://www.cureparkinsons.org.uk
http://www.parkinsonsmovement.com

Made in the USA
Charleston, SC
09 May 2013